Introduction

THERE is no shortage of evidence that psychiatric illness is very common in the community. It has been estimated that between 10% and 20% of the general practitioner's practice population are mentally or emotionally disturbed (Shepherd et al., 1966). Studies of attending patients have shown that up to one third of patients at general practice surgeries have some form of psychological disturbance, though not necessarily psychiatric disease (Goldberg and Blackwell, 1970; Hoeper et al., 1979; Skuse and Williams, 1984; Wright and Perini, 1987). Despite the constraints of limited consulting time, most of these patients are managed within general practice without referral to a psychiatrist.

People who seek medical help for these symptoms generally turn first to their general practitioner. The commonest psychiatric illness seen by general practitioners is depression and this is also one of the commonest clinical illness found in attending patients. Surveys have shown that 1 in 10 attending patients can be diagnosed as suffering from depression and 1 in 20 would meet criteria for major depressive disorder (Blacker and Clare, 1987). Depressive illness seen by general practitioners is not trivial or transitory and about half of the patients with the disorder are unable to continue with their normal lives (Johnson and Mellor, 1977). This depression is not weakness of character but a clearly differentiated clinical illness like diabetes or hypertension. It is potentially life threatening as most of the 4000 suicides in the UK each year suffered from depression. Though depression can now be treated effectively it is clear that many sufferers do not receive the treatment that they desperately need. The recognition and diagnosis of depression is important, as it is a treatable disease and most depressed patients can be fully and effectively managed in general practice.

The cost of depression

Depression is not only a painful and distressing illness for patients and their carers, it is a costly problem for the National Health Service in terms of frequent consultations with general practitioners and sometimes inappropriate investigations or referrals (Croft-Jeffries and Wilkinson, 1989). Depression causes prolonged absence from work or poor work performance and there are economic consequences for both patients and society.

The Mental Health Foundation (Thompson and Pudney, 1990) estimates that in 1989 over 71 million working days were lost in Britain because of mental illness including depression. This amounts to 17% of all sickness absences from work and cost the country £4 billion in lost working days and the NHS £6.8 million for treatment.

The cost of depression is summarized in Table 1.

Table 1 *The cost of depression*

Patient	Painful and distressing especially if unrecognized
	May worsen the effects of physical illness
	Loss of work (psychiatric illnesses last many months)
Family	Very stressful to manage illness in the community
Society	Prolonged absence from work
	Poor work performance
NHS	Frequent consultations in general practice
	Some inappropriate investigations
	Some inappropriate specialist referrals
Doctor	Managing patients can be stressful

The general practitioner's role in management

It is widely accepted that the general practitioner, who has a continuous relationship with patients and families, is well placed to manage psychiatric illness in the community since presenting conditions are often a mix of physical, psychological and social elements.

1. Many patients with psychiatric disturbance do not consider themselves in need of care and would not attend a psychiatrist.

2. Physical and mental illness often co-exist.

3. Many psychiatric disorders are family affairs in that they are connected with family problems and are best understood when viewed against this background.

4. General practitioners are available to the patient at his next relapse, when a junior psychiatrist has often moved on.

Some of the differences of approach to managing depression are due to the fact that general practitioners deal with a different population of psychiatrically ill people who have different needs from hospital inpatients or day patients (all of whom have already been screened by a general practitioner). The general practitioner also sees the early stage of the disease in patients who are eventually referred to a psychiatrist.

There is a strong direct relationship between depression and physical disease. Some patients seem to be particularly susceptible to both physical and psychiatric illness and the secondary effect of chronic pain is a further handicap and strain on a patient's natural resistance to psychiatric illness. Depression commonly accompanies alcohol problems, bereavement and childbirth for which general practitioners are commonly consulted.

General practitioners are now considered as a main source of help for depressed people rather than the church or the extended family. Depression is now much more accepted as an illness and this has certainly led to a greater number of cases being reported.

DEPRESSION

RECOGNITION AND MANAGEMENT IN GENERAL PRACTICE

BY

ALASTAIR F WRIGHT MD, FRCGP

Published by

The Royal College of General Practitioners

1993

The Royal College of General Practitioners was founded in 1952, with this object:

"To encourage, foster and maintain the highest possible standards in general medical practice and for that purpose to take or join with others in taking steps consistent with the charitable nature of that object which may assist towards the same."

Among its responsibilities under its Royal Charter the College is entitled to:

"Diffuse information on all matters affecting general medical practice and issue such publications as may assist the object of the College."

First edition 1988
Second edition 1992

Published by the Royal College of General Practitioners

Typeset by Exe Valley Dataset Ltd, Exeter, Devon

Printed by Hillprint Ltd, Bishop Auckland, Co. Durham.

ISBN 0 85084 180 1

Contents

Acknowledgement

The Editor of the Clinical Series is grateful to Duphar Laboratories Ltd for assistance in publishing this booklet

A patient information audio cassette
'Coping with Depression' by Dr Alastair Wright
is available from Duphar Laboratories Ltd
Telephone: 0703 470284

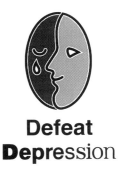

**Defeat
Depression**

A National Campaign organised by the Royal College of Psychiatrists
in association with the Royal College of General Practitioners

Further information on the Defeat Depression Campaign is available from
the Campaign Office, Royal College of Psychiatrists, 17 Belgrave Square, London SW1X 8PG
Telephone: 071 235 2351   Facsimile: 071 245 1231

"If depression is one of the commonest conditions that general practitioners see, if it is possible to diagnose it by fairly simple questions and by listening, if it is eminently treatable and patients do get better with treatment, is it not a major clinical priority for doctors in the front line of the health service?"

Denis Pereira Gray

What is depression?

DEPRESSION is an unsatisfactory term, since it can describe an everyday mood, a symptom, or a disease. The older terms, 'melancholia' or 'neurasthenia' are more descriptive and it is worthwhile remembering them when considering depression as they add important emphasis to our concepts of the clinical picture. Feeling depressed is not the same thing as having depression.

Major depressive disorder

Research psychiatrists have found it useful to define a syndrome of 'Major depressive disorder' (APA, 1987) which is useful for research work and valuable in assessing antidepressant treatment. Major depressive disorder is seen and treated in general practice but use of the term does not imply that other forms of depression are trivial. Minor depression of mood may or may not go on to become major depressive disorder and there are many grey tones of mood disorders in between.

Other types of depression are also important in general practice, such as milder depressive episodes which do not reach the thresholds for major depression and mixed anxiety/depression states which are commonly seen in the community. Every practice has some patients who appear to have a depressive personality and suffer lifelong mild fluctuating depression (dysthymia) punctuated by occasional major depressive episodes which are superimposed. Some patients may show atypical features or have depression associated with multiple somatic complaints. In general practice the boundary between depressive illness and anxiety disorders is not clear and mixed states are common. Anxiety symptoms are common in depression and, if they are dramatic, may mask the depression. Many depressed patients are wrongly diagnosed, and treated, as anxiety states.

An important subtype is the depression associated with dramatic mood swings into euphoria or hypomania. This type is now often called 'bipolar disorder' in preference to manic depressive illness. This term is intended to include patients who have *ever* had a manic syndrome, whether or not they have been depressed. 'Unipolar' is intended to mean people who have been depressed but never manic.

Causes

Depressive illness has a variety of causes of which familial and genetic factors are important. It often occurs at times of psychosocial transition such as adolescence, marriage, childbirth or the onset of old age; major stressful life events and losses; through lack of social support; and concurrent physical illness, all of which increase vulnerability.

The neurochemical basis of depression is uncertain. The currently most popular hypothesis suggests that the disease is due to reduced availability of 5-hydroxytryptamine (5HT) at the synapses as antidepressant drugs are thought to act on 5HT and noradrenergic receptors. Other theories of causation implicate noradrenaline or melatonin owing to the seasonal variation in depression in some patients (seasonal affective disorder) and to the diurnal changes in symptoms. The relatively high prevalence of depression in women and the special risk of depression in the puerperium suggest a hormonal cause. While this sounds plausible, there does not appear to be good research evidence to support this theory.

Life stresses such as childbirth or the menopause are associated with vulnerability to depression but the clinical features of depressive illness in these patients are no different from those in which there is no such precipitating factor. Most researchers report that less than 10% of those suffering significant life stresses actually become depressed, suggesting that personality factors are important in vulnerability. Conversely, hypomanic episodes in bipolar depression can be precipitated by life stresses and the view that severe so called endogenous depression had no precipitant causes has been shown to be incorrect.

Clinical picture

Depression is a serious, potentially fatal illness which must not be underestimated. Thoughts of suicide or death are common and self-esteem is low. The symptoms are severe and persistent and often associated with changes in sleep pattern, libido, appetite and weight.

The crucial feature of all types of depression is the lowering of mood often accompanied by tearfulness. The depressed patient has a painful inability to experience pleasure (anhedonia) and has marked impairment of concentration. While the patient may not complain of or even notice this loss, family members will be well aware of the change in his or her behaviour. Withdrawal from family and friends is common as is neglect of activities that were previously a source of pleasure. Slowed thinking, indecisiveness and problems with concentration are common and the patient may complain of difficulty remembering things as a consequence of this loss of concentration. In almost all cases there is a characteristic way of thinking with persistent negative attitudes and thoughts of personal worthlessness. The smallest task may seem difficult or impossible to the patient, who has an unrealistically poor evaluation of his or her own worth. Excessive guilt may be felt about past actions or in relation to perceived shortcomings. Extreme pessimism about the future contributes to suicide risk.

Although the pervasive mood disorder of disquiet, morbid restlessness and malaise is usually a main feature of the disease, there are many other additional features. These include loss of energy and interest; inhibition of thought, drive and initiative; irritability and sleep disturbance with early morning wakening. Patients frequently have feelings of helplessness and hopelessness and suicidal ideation. They show disturbed appetite, weight and sexual functions and a whole variety of satellite somatic symptoms.

Patients' descriptions

Patients may describe the onset of depression as falling into a black well from which there is no escape. Others say that they feel that the sun has gone out or that they feel trapped in a green bottle separate from the rest of humanity, unable to love or be loved. Doctors who have experienced both physical disease and depressive illness describe the anguish of depression as being greater than the pain of myocardial infarction and much less easy to relieve.

The distress of being depressed may be made worse for the patient by the stigma still attached to mental health problems. Even in 1991 a public attitude survey (MORI, 1992) carried out in several different locations in England demonstrated the prevailing view that psychiatric illness implied inherent abnormality, weakness and instability. One doctor recognizing that "Depression is very much an illness ..." could describe his "desperate unhappiness" and admit "... it feels different, one feels stigmatized ..." (Anon, 1989). Despite a more open attitude to discussing such illnesses and the broadcast accounts of their depressive illness by several well known and successful public figures, depression is frequently linked to the ill person's inability to cope with life. Depressed patients need to be reassured by their doctor that depression is not weakness of character but a well defined clinical illness.

Natural history of depression

The normal course and outcome of depression in general practice is not clearly established as there is great variation in the results of different research reports. Sometimes there is a lack of specification of which disorders are being analysed or a great variation in the severity of the illness of patients in the same analysis groups. The follow-up groups chosen are often very different, as is the length of follow-up. Finally, it is important to distinguish between acute, short-lived episodes and more chronic illness. Patients with chronic depressive illness tend to have high attendance rates and contribute substantially to overall general practitioner workload.

What is clear is that depression seen in general practice is a very common and often severe condition which causes much misery and distress to patients and their families. Most patients can be adequately treated in general practice without referral provided the treating doctor is prepared to provide support and regular, systematic follow-up of progress and compliance with treatment. The prognosis for adequately treated patients is good.

The need for comprehensive and systematic research work in this area is urgent. Teaching on the recognition and management of depression in the community should be based on research and experience using representative community samples rather than hospital inpatients or outpatient samples. Research work done in inner city areas convenient to academic departments may not be typical of experience throughout general practice.

Severity

Depressive illness seen in general practice is commonly said to be milder, more reactive and less biological than depression seen by psychiatrists. In practice it is not uncommon to see patients who are more severely depressed but are not referred for a variety of reasons or who will not accept referral to a psychiatrist. This latter problem has been eased by more

psychiatrists becoming attached to health centres and seeing patients there, so avoiding the stigma for patients of attending a mental hospital.

The traditional view that the more severely depressed patients are all likely to be referred and managed by a consultant is more true of patients suffering from psychotic illness. While many severely depressed patients are rightly referred for specialist help, referral of depressed patients is often made on the basis of additional complicating factors such as:

- personality difficulties
- alcohol abuse
- non-response to treatment
- danger of suicide
- patient request for referral
- family pressure for admission.

A good prognosis

Mann et al. (1981), in a prospective study of 93 patients with non-psychotic illness in two Warwickshire practices, showed that a third improved within the first 6 months, a third ran a variable intermittent course, and a third had chronic persistent symptoms. Relatively few prospective studies have been published on the course and outcome of depression. Johnson and Mellor (1977) found that 69% of patients recovered after 4 months and a further 10% improved. Widmer and Cadoret (1979) in the USA demonstrated that only 13% of their depressed patients had suffered episodes lasting longer than 2 years and that the median episode length was 4 months. Dunn and Skuse (1981) showed that women are particularly prone to recurrence of depression and less likely to make a full recovery.

Social factors do play a part in chronicity but the main predictive factor appears to be severity of the disease at onset. The patient's perception of quality of social life is also an important prognostic indicator particularly as regards marriage and family life.

The relatively small number of patients who become chronically depressed can be seriously handicapped as a result. Freeling et al. (1985) have shown that recognized cases do best even when they do not comply with treatment. Chronicity of depression in primary care may be something to do with non-detection and therefore non-treatment of existing cases by general practitioners.

Making a diagnosis

Many of the symptoms of depression are very common and are shared with a variety of physical diseases so that there may be a problem with diagnosis, especially if patients present with the somatic rather than the psychological features of the illness. Individual symptoms are of little help in diagnosis if considered in isolation, though the two symptoms of anhedonia and loss of concentration are important diagnostically because they are relatively specific.

It is vital to consider the whole clinical picture, making a positive diagnosis based on symptoms and behaviour and not simply on the basis of exclusion. It is never safe to label a patient as depressed simply because his or her symptoms do not fit neatly into any common physical syndrome.

The problems of identifying depression in attending patients are dealt with more fully in a later chapter (4).

2

Clinical subtypes

THERE are various ways of categorizing illness depending on the purpose of the categorization. In clinical practice the purpose of classification is to help identification, determine appropriate treatment and to predict progress and outcome. Listing subtypes of depression based on aetiological, symptomatic or other criteria is of little clinical utility. Similarly, subdivision into endogenous or reactive, neurotic or psychotic subtypes is of more value for research and administration than for clinical work. In the community it is more serviceable to think in terms of severity and to consider whether there are associated problems such as manic features, alcohol abuse, personality disorder or serious physical illness.

It is worthwhile clinically to think of depression in terms of psychosocial transitions such as adolescence, marriage, childbirth, the menopause or bereavement. Thinking of the special features of depressive illness at different ages has the advantage of increasing the doctor's awareness of the possibility of depression which may not present directly.

Depression becomes more common with increasing age but it occurs in children as well as the aged. It is more frequently diagnosed in women than men and appears to be more widespread in young men, at least in the USA, than was formerly recognized. There are now substantial ethnic minority groups in the UK and doctors should be aware that in some cultures depression may present a somewhat different clinical picture with patients more likely to express their distress in somatic terms. For example, there is some evidence that Asian patients are more likely to present somatic symptoms and have more intense expressions of shame.

Depression in children, in adolescents and in the elderly may be recognized in differing ways.

Childhood and adolescence

The possibility of depression in a disturbed child is often missed because it is not considered. Children suffer depressed mood just as adults do but children do not often complain or are unable to verbalize their feelings. Delayed depressive reactions and behaviour disturbances can occur in children who have been sexually abused and this possibility should be remembered by health professionals.

In addition to depressed mood and even suicidal thoughts the child may show features of anxiety or irritability and have disturbed sleep. They may refuse school and develop phobias or hypochondriasis and they often show obsessional personality features. Their school performance often deteriorates with the onset of the illness and unexplained abdominal pain is common. Antidepressant drugs can often be used with advantage.

General practitioners may be reluctant to diagnose depressive illness in adolescents as adolescent turmoil with low self-esteem is common in this age group. Adolescents do develop full blown depressive illness resulting in much misery and lowered self-image. They more often look depressed than do children but they too often find it difficult to explain to the doctor how they feel. Interaction with peers and adults is frequently quite markedly disturbed resulting in problems at school or college. Low levels of interest and concentration can result in unexpectedly poor performance in examinations and this can be a valuable clue to depressive illness.

Adolescents respond just as satisfactorily to treatment as do adults.

The elderly

Recognition of depression in elderly people can be particularly difficult for a number of reasons. Older people may feel that their depressed mood is a normal part of ageing and may not seek help for their depression. Many believe they should consult a doctor for physical complaints only and may also be less likely to accept psychological explanations for their symptoms.

Estimates of the prevalence of depression vary depending on the diagnostic criteria used but probably at any one time 10–15% of people over 65 suffer from significant depressive illness with higher rates among attending patients. The work of Williamson et al. (1964) in the 1960s suggested that most of the diagnosable psychiatric morbidity in elderly patients was not recognized by their general practitioner. This research has subsequently been much criticized, especially with regard to the detection of dementia by general practitioners, and a number of their findings have not been confirmed by later work. More recent work by MacDonald (1986) suggested that the London general practitioners studied *overdiagnosed* depression but then paradoxically failed to treat it appropriately. Most research shows that depression in older patients generally responds well to treatment though there is also some evidence that the elderly are somewhat less responsive and that the prognosis is less good. Extra care is required when adjusting dosage of antidepressant drugs as these patients are more susceptible to drug side-effects. It is regrettable that elderly depressed patients do not always receive the treatment likely to improve the quality of their lives.

Rather than seeming depressed, older people may appear to be complaining, querulous, difficult and demanding. They may complain of feeling 'empty' or 'cold inside' rather than saying they are miserable or depressed. Both they and the doctor may attribute symptoms of depression to co-existing physical illness. Chronic somatic disease may precipitate depressive illness just as self-neglect in elderly depressed patients may result in physical illness.

If an elderly depressed patient is confused, forgetful or withdrawn, he or she may be regarded as demented and be denied appropriate treatment for the real problem of depression. Depression develops relatively quickly, dementia insidiously. Depressed patients appear more distressed and less blunted than those with dementia. They are guilty, self-reproachful and often have somatic symptoms which are uncommon in dementia. It is very important to distinguish between the two as response to treatment is much better in depression. In doubtful cases a trial of treatment is worthwhile.

Wilkin and Williams (1986) remind us that physical ageing is accompanied by a decline in social functioning and a gradual limitation of various activities of daily living. Psychological ageing accompanies these biological and social processes making the old person less able to cope with change in circumstances and emotional problems. These age-related processes must be understood when deciding what is normal (Williams, 1993). Increasing age, physical illness and social isolation are all associated with an increased likelihood of depression. The general practitioner who knows his or her patients is well placed to deal with the problems which may arise.

The new contract for general practice in April 1990 introduced mandatory screening of people over 75 by the primary care team and it seems likely that this will improve the detection of depression and dementia. Depression should be remembered in the list of factors to be screened for. The contract does not contain guidelines for practice teams but the Royal College of General Practitioners is publishing recommendations for health checks for people aged 75 and over (Williams and Wallace, 1993). The general practitioner should consider having his own at-risk register and occasional home visiting is important for these patients.

It is most important that, having made the diagnosis, the doctor does something about it (Williamson et al., 1964). Depression in old people responds to the same drugs and interventions that are effective in younger patients. Electro-convulsive therapy may have a useful place in severe cases, some psychiatrists considering it safer in these circumstances than psychotropic drugs.

Clues to depression in the elderly are listed in Table 2.

Table 2 *Clues to depression in the elderly*

- A history of recent deterioration in functioning
- Distressing life events, for example bereavement, having to leave home, painful physical disease
- Expressions of guilt or despair
- A past history of depression or a family history of depression or mania

---

Postnatal depression

The clinical picture is similar to depression at other stages of life but the illness is even less understandable to patients, occurring as it does at a time normally of great joy to mother, father and the family. Depressive feelings of guilt, inability to cope and hopelessness are focused on the patient's role as a mother. The inability to feel normal emotions and react appropriately to the baby affect the bonding process between mother and newborn baby and this effect may be lifelong. In this way, the child itself may have an increased vulnerability to depression in adult life in addition to any genetic susceptibility.

When the symptoms are mild the patient may be treated at home providing careful supervision is practicable. It is important that mother and baby are not separated as this exacerbates the effect on bonding and the sense of uselessness felt by the mother. When there are psychotic features (puerperal psychosis) admission is mandatory as both mother and baby are at risk of physical harm if the mother suffers delusions. Ideally, admission should be to a mother and baby unit. Whether given at home or hospital the treatment should be energetic if much suffering is to be avoided.

Dysthymia

Dysthymia is defined in the DSM-IIIR, an American list of diagnostic criteria increasingly quoted in this country (APA, 1987). It is an American term for an important condition which, like depression, may go unrecognized and is one of the explanations of 'frequent attenders' in the general practitioner's consulting room. The clinical picture is of a chronic disturbance of mood and associated symptoms which are not of sufficient severity and duration to justify a diagnosis of major depressive disorder. Patients have little interest or pleasure in most or all their usual activities or pastimes. They normally function quite well at work and in their social contacts but are more likely to abuse medicaments and be high users of general practitioner services. The cardinal feature of the condition is *chronicity* rather than severity and patients are sometimes diagnosed as 'depressive personality'.

This diagnosis should be considered when the symptoms have been present for a long time and are less severe than in major depression or when major depression has been in *partial* remission for a period of two years. The possibility should be remembered when dealing with 'difficult' patients, patients with a 'fat file', or those thought to have a dependent personality. Predisposing factors are chronic physical disorder, chronic psychosocial stresses and the presence of another mental disorder.

Atypical depression

Psychiatrists have recently been using this term to describe depressed patients who show symptoms of overeating and oversleeping with paradoxical worsening of anxiety and irritability in the evening. The syndrome is not common but is important as the unusual symptom pattern means that the diagnosis is liable to be missed and the patients labelled as 'worried well' or personality disordered. Monoamine-oxidase inhibitors (MAOIs) have been shown to be beneficial and are probably to be preferred to the tricyclic antidepressants (Casey, 1990).

Bipolar disorder (manic depression)

Most practices will have a number of patients who suffer from depressive episodes which are associated with dramatic swings in mood through hypomania to overt mania with pressure of speech, grandiose ideas and loss of normal social inhibitions. Control of this distressing condition has been much improved by the relatively recent introduction of lithium salts in maintenance treatment, though the beneficial therapeutic effects of lithium have long been recognized (Cade, 1949). Lithium has a mood-regulating action and is specific in this condition. Dosage is controlled by serial blood sampling which can be done simply within the practice.

Agitated depression

It is important to remember that depressed patients may show marked agitation, anxiety and apprehension. Appropriate treatment is with an antidepressant drug from the sedative group and *not* benzodiazepine anxiolytics, which on their own may be harmful and carry a high risk of developing dependence. It is sometimes difficult to distinguish agitated depression from episodes of acute anxiety in patients who are adjusting after a dramatic incident or other emotional shock. They have more normal reactivity of mood than those suffering from depressive illness.

Bereavement depression

Grief following the death of a loved one is a universal human experience and should not be medicalized by the prescription of benzodiazepine anxiolytics except when symptoms are disabling. These drugs are often not requested by the bereaved person but, inappropriately, by the family carers. They can worsen the normal dazed and numb feelings, affect memory and long-term use may cause dependence. Inappropriate drug therapy in stress-related disorders can inhibit patients' own efforts to organize themselves to adjust to their changed circumstances (Lader, 1975).

Most bereaved people pass through a short period of acute reaction when they feel dazed and numb and follow their normal activities in a reflex, automatic manner; they often have poor subsequent memory of this stage. Within weeks or even days of this phase most people have depressive symptoms such as disturbed sleep and appetite, weeping and depressed mood without necessarily developing full blown depressive illness. Most bereaved individuals come slowly to accept the death of their loved one and readjust but in some, depressive illness will supervene and they will require antidepressant therapy. A few will be unable to readjust and may, for example, be unable to dispose of the clothes and belongings of the deceased partner. These patients usually respond better to a behavioural approach rather than to antidepressants.

3

How common is depression?

THERE is no doubt that psychiatric illness is common in the community and that general practitioners see many patients who are depressed. Estimates of incidence and prevalence of depression and of mental illness in general will vary depending on diagnostic criteria and the methods used to detect cases. Nevertheless, it is probably true that as many as 1 in 3 general practice consultations have a demonstrable psychosocial component, though not necessarily involving psychiatric illness, while about 1 in 7 people experience some of the symptoms of depression in one year. A substantially greater number will experience an episode of 'depressive disorder' at some time during their lifetime.

Prevalence of mental illness

An important source of information on the prevalence of psychiatric illness seen by general practitioners in this country is the pioneering work of Professor Michael Shepherd and his colleagues at the Institute of Psychiatry General Practice Research Unit. From a relatively largescale study, Shepherd et al. (1966) showed that 14% of general practitioner patients consulted at least once each year for a condition diagnosed as entirely or largely psychiatric and that half these conditions had been present for at least a year. Only 1 in 20 (5%) of these identified patients had seen a psychiatrist in the study year. Several workers have since confirmed frank psychiatric illness in between 20% and 25% of attending patients (Goldberg, 1972, 1985; Sims and Salmons, 1975).

Bridges and Goldberg (1985) using the DSM-III criteria studied nearly 500 patients in the Manchester area attending their general practitioner with a new illness. Thirty-three per cent satisfied the criteria for psychiatric illness, 13% for adjustment disorders (stress disorders), and only 54% had purely physical illness.

More recently Goldberg and Huxley (1992), from their work in the Greater Manchester area, have estimated annual period prevalence rates for mental illness (whether recognized or not) counting people who are ill for at least 2 weeks in the calendar year. For every 1000 patients at risk in the community, they estimate that 315 have mental illness, 230 seek medical help, 23 are referred to secondary care, and only 6 become inpatients.

Defining a 'case'

Research psychiatrists (Williams et al., 1980; Kendell, 1988) have devoted much effort in trying to define 'caseness', in other words the point at which a set of symptoms become clinically significant, for example when depressive symptoms become a recognizable depressive disorder. Instruments for measuring symptoms do exist both for patient-completed questionnaires and standardized interviews.

Structured interviews define the questions to be asked and the way they are to be asked is laid down in advance (Hamilton, 1960; Goldberg et al., 1970; Dean et al., 1983). Written definitions are provided for each item. These interview schedules are generally unsuitable for use by general practitioners as they are inflexible and training (standardization) is needed to achieve consistent results. More recent, simpler standardized instruments (Lewis et al., 1989) may prove of practical value in general practice.

One relatively simple scale, the Montgomery Asberg Depression Rating Scale (MADRS) (Montgomery and Asberg, 1979), has become popular and may have a place as an *aide-mémoire* for general practitioners in following the progress of a patient's symptoms and the effectiveness of treatment as the questionnaire is said to be very sensitive to change.

Self-assessment questionnaires eliminate interview bias and can be used to estimate levels of psychiatric pathology in populations or to screen patients for psychological disturbance. These patient-completed questionnaires, for example the General Health Questionnaire (Goldberg, 1978, 1986) or the Hospital Anxiety and Depression Scale (Zigmond and Snaith, 1983), are generally acceptable to patients, do not require extra consultation time and deserve wider trial by general practitioners in routine clinical work (Overton and Wise, 1980; Robins et al., 1984; Wright and Perini, 1987).

Even using these methods, differing prevalence rates can be explained by:

● the way symptoms are elicited

● the choice of measuring instrument

● the cut-off score for caseness.

Attitudes of research psychiatrists are also changing with regard to measuring caseness. Instead of simply counting the number of symptoms complained of by the patient, more emphasis is now placed on the type of symptoms, their severity, statistical relationships and the help-seeking behaviour shown by the patient.

The division of depressive disorder into endogenous or reactive subgroups is now becoming outdated and more emphasis is placed on the form and degree of the depressive reaction than to the circumstances against which it arose.

General practitioner workload

Buchan and Richardson (1973) have shown that general practice patients attending with psychiatric illness not only have more consultations but that consultations with such patients take longer than average.

It is difficult to separate workload due to new cases of illness from that due to chronic illness. In my own practice a random sample of 96 attending women was followed-up using the General Health Questionnaire and repeating the test in one year (Wright, 1988). Mean consultation rates were 13.2 for chronic patients whose test remained abnormal compared with 6.2 for patients with two normal tests and 8.0 for patients becoming ill during the year. Figures for men were similar but somewhat lower. In the same practice a study of incidence showed 125 suspected new cases of psychiatric illness in one year with 111 confirmed by psychological testing suggesting two new cases per week for one doctor (Wright, 1990).

The proportion of new case workload due to depression is estimated by Barber (1981) at about four new cases of depressive illness per doctor per month. A major component in workload is that arising from the management of recurring or chronic depressive illness and there is also evidence (Widmer and Cadoret, 1978) for a marked rise in patient-initiated contacts *prior* to the diagnosis of depression. Studies of subsequent developing depression showed that the median interval between episodes of recurrent depression was three years and that 30% of depressed patients had a recurrence within seven years (Widmer and Cadoret, 1979).

Prevalence of depression

Depression is the commonest psychiatric illness seen by general practitioners; in fact, it is one of the commonest clinical problems that general practitioners have to deal with.

Prevalence rates for depression in general practice, based on standardized interview, vary considerably between studies (Casey et al., 1984; Robins et al., 1984) probably owing to differences in research method rather than true interpractice variation. Analysis of the results of a number of studies suggest that about 5% of consulting patients show major depression, another 5% milder episodes, and a further 10% will have some depressive symptoms (Blacker and Clare, 1987). This means that, on average, at least one depressed patient will be seen at every consulting session. Most depression is therefore treated in general practice with probably less than 10% of patients being referred to specialist psychiatric services.

Associated factors

Sociodemographic

The experience of any individual general practitioner in managing depression and his ability to recognize the illness may be biased by the age/sex distribution of his patients and the social class make-up of his practice. Research done in individual practices may report sociodemographic associations which simply reflect the peculiarities of the practice population served. Nevertheless, there are clear relationships between depressive illness and age, sex and socio-economic class. Findings of association between depression and marital status tend to be difficult to interpret but it seems to be that marriage increases the risk of depression in women and decreases the risk in men!

Age

The clinical picture of depressive illness can be different at different ages. For example, depression in children can be manifest in school refusal, phobias and alimentary disorders while adolescents may have very marked disturbances of behaviour. Old people may talk of feeling 'empty' or 'cold inside' rather than feeling 'depressed'.

Sex

Most studies show many more women than men diagnosed as suffering from depression. This difference is real and there is probably a 2:1 female/male ratio. However, it should also be remembered that women are known to seek medical care more readily and to consult more for minor complaints of all kinds. Men are less likely to consult and some may also express their depression in less socially acceptable ways such as by alcohol abuse or violent behaviour. Also men are more likely to be labelled 'personality disorder'.

Two studies in 1984 both reported the usual excess of depression in women and alcoholism and personality disorder in men but found that the prevalence of *total* psychiatric disorder was the same in both sexes (Casey et al., 1984; Robins et al., 1984). In my own practice there was no statistically significant difference between men and women in total GHQ-28 score while the diagnostic labels applied were strikingly different in the two sexes as was the prescribing of psychotropic drugs (Wright, 1988).

Women are said to be less likely to recover completely than men and so are more likely to become chronic. In practices with a large number of middle-aged women this 'gathering' effect will show as a higher than average prevalence in cross-sectional studies unless chronicity is controlled for. From the large study from the National Institute for Mental Health in the USA it appears that young adults now seem more likely to develop major depression and more likely to consult their general practitioner when they do so (Robins et al., 1984).

Socio-economic status

There is some evidence that patients who have had higher education are less likely to develop depression than the lower social classes. Patients of higher social class are more able to verbalize their symptoms and are probably more efficient at obtaining suitable medical care. Studying 572 women in London, Brown and Harris (1978) suggested that depression in their series of patients was caused primarily by psychosocial factors. It would be harmful to patients if general practitioners misinterpreted this work and regarded depression as a social disease to be treated mainly by social management. Jenkins and Shepherd (1983), reviewing the extensive research data on minor psychiatric morbidity, concluded that the role of social factors in depressive illness is complex and poorly understood.

4

Recognizing depression in the community

GENERAL practitioners are faced with a bewildering range and variety of continuously changing emotional states which do not fit the neat categories set out in the existing glossaries and classifications, which are largely based on experience with psychiatric inpatients. A further difficulty is the need to be aware of patients at risk who would not fulfil psychiatric diagnostic criteria and to be concerned with patients who do not present directly, for example mothers of apparently well children who are brought too frequently with catarrh or colds. Mothers may be poor copers because of depression. What is important in depression, irrespective of cause or subtype, is to realize that it is eminently treatable and that it is worthwhile to identify patients who are clinically depressed, to relieve their suffering, shorten the course of the illness and try to prevent recurrence.

Classification of psychiatric illness

The two most widely used classifications of psychiatric illness are the World Heath Organization's International Classification of Disease (WHO, 1978) and the Diagnostic and Statistical Manual of Mental Disorders of the American Psychiatric Association (1987). The International Classification of Disease presents a menu of choices for diagnosis but the rubrics are skewed towards severe or psychotic disorders and are weak in minor disorders seen frequently in general practice. In the latest revision (ICD-10) modifications are being made to increase its usefulness in the community and some definition of terms is now available. The American manual uses an alternative approach which aims to define each condition, presenting recipes rather than a menu. These classifications are too bulky for table-top use but the desk-top computer is changing all this and automatic coding using the standard Read codes (Chisholm, 1990) is already available on some practice management computer systems.

Major depressive disorder

The DSM-IIIR defines depression in terms 'major' depressive disorder (Table 3). To meet the diagnostic criteria for this condition there must be persistent dysphoric mood and at least four from a list of major symptoms present for at least two weeks. The DSM-IIIR allows multi-axial classification and has an axis specifically for personality disorder. Personality factors are important in the onset and diagnosis of depression.

This DSM-IIIR definition is useful particularly in research work and especially in assessing the effectiveness of treatment but the term 'major' does not imply that other forms of depression are not significant. Major depressive disorder is seen in general practice but other, milder forms of depression are also important and mixed anxiety and depression is common. These types of depression have already been detailed in Chapter 2.

Clinical classification

Formal definitions of depressive disorder depend largely on the number and severity of symptoms whereas general practitioners are also guided by sociodemographic or family factors and social stresses or supports. These non-symptomatic factors are important in

Table 3 *DSM diagnostic criteria for major depressive episode*

A. Dysphoric mood or loss of interest or pleasure in all or almost all usual activities and pastimes. The dysphoric mood is characterized by symptoms such as the following: depressed, sad, blue, hopeless, low, down in the dumps, irritable. The mood disturbance must be prominent and relatively persistent, but not necessarily the most dominant symptom, and does not include momentary shifts from one dysphoric mood to another dysphoric mood, for example anxiety to depression to anger, such as are seen in states of acute psychotic turmoil. (For children under six, dysphoric mood may have to be inferred from a persistently sad facial expression.)

B. At least four of the following symptoms have each been present nearly every day for a period of at least two weeks (in children under six, at least three of the first four):

   1. Poor appetite or significant weight loss (when not dieting) or increased appetite or significant weight gain (in children under six, consider failure to make expected weight gains).

   2. Insomnia or hypersomnia.

   3. Psychomotor agitation or retardation (but not merely subjective feelings of restlessness or being slowed down), (in children under six, hypoactivity).

   4. Loss of interest or pleasure in usual activities, or decrease in sexual drive not limited to a period when delusional or hallucinating (in children under six, signs of apathy).

   5. Loss of energy; fatigue.

   6. Feelings of worthlessness, self-reproach, or excessive or inappropriate guilt (either may be delusional).

   7. Complaints or evidence of diminished ability to think or concentrate, such as slowed thinking, or indecisiveness not associated with marked loosening of associations or incoherence.

   8. Recurrent thoughts of death, suicidal ideation, wishes to be dead, or suicide attempt.

Source: American Psychiatric Association, Task Force on Nomenclature and Statistics (1980) *Diagnostic and Statistical Manual of Mental Disorders.* 3rd edn. Washington DC, APA.

clinical decision making and management but are very difficult to measure or standardize. Attitudes of research psychiatrists have also changed with regard to measuring caseness. Instead of focusing on the number of symptoms complained of, more emphasis is now placed on the type of symptoms, their severity, statistical relationships and the help-seeking behaviour shown by patients. While most general practitioners do not record diagnoses in the terms familiar to research psychiatrists, many think of diagnosis in physical, psychological and social terms using labels that their patients can understand.

The main aim in general practice is to recognize and treat depression at an early stage so it is less suitable to think in terms of exclusive criteria. In practice many general practitioners tend to evolve their own methods of classification and to use working labels rather than formal diagnoses. These working diagnoses may be vague and can be criticized as simply 'justifying treatment' but the same criticism can be applied not only in psychiatry but in other branches of medicine. Working labels are sufficient clinically if they can be linked to effective treatment and make sense to the patient.

The purpose of diagnosis is to predict treatment and outcome but unfortunately the value of psychiatric diagnosis in this context is limited and diagnoses vary greatly between doctor and doctor (Kendell, 1975). Indeed some iconoclasts (Marinker, 1973) go so far as to maintain that psychiatric diagnosis is the justification for treatment rather than the reason for it. Balint (1964) takes the following view on psychiatric labels: "At best they are diagnoses of symptoms, not of illnesses. Their limited usefulness remains unchanged even if these diagnostic labels change according to the prevalent fashion in psychiatry."

Working labels are, however, essential in planning the management of an individual patient and in practice one must consider not only the diagnostic label but make an assessment of the patient's personality and circumstances including social stresses and supports.

Inappropriate labels

Some labels are inappropriate, however, especially if their use leads to patients being denied treatment.

Some older general practitioners may have been taught ideas on psychiatry derived from study of the 10% of patients who see psychiatrists and the 1% who are admitted to hospital rather than the 90% who never see a specialist. The traditional distinction between 'endogenous' and 'reactive' depressions is of little practical significance in terms of severity, outcome and likely response to anti-depressants. Most psychiatrists have now abandoned this distinction and concentrate on the extent and severity of the depressive disorder rather than the circumstances against which it developed. General practitioners who classify patients by whether or not their depression is 'understandable' to the doctor can deprive their patients of the relief of antidepressant drug therapy.

Patients may also be wrongly labelled 'anxiety state' if there is a marked anxiety component to their symptoms. Despite the fact that research has shown that depressive illness is one of the commonest conditions in general practice, prescribing rates for antidepressants are relatively low and patients are still pre-scribed benzodiazepines inappropriately.

Clinical features of depression

It is useful to summarize the clinical features of the depression seen in general practice under mood, changed thinking and physio-logical symptoms (Table 4).

Aids to diagnosing depression

Many of the symptoms of depression are so common that if taken alone they are of little value for diagnosis or in predicting outcome. Other symptoms, such as psychomotor retard-ation or excessive guilt, are very diagnostic but are so rare in general practice that they are of little use in most cases.

Table 4 *Clinical features of depression*

Changed mood
Persistent sadness
Pathological pessimism
Abnormal self-reproach
Lassitude
Inability to feel
Thoughts of suicide
Weeping
Shame

Changed drive and thinking
Unable to cope
Loss of interest and concentration
Difficulty in making decisions
Hopeless and helpless
Wish to escape

Physical symptoms
Tired all the time
Aches and pains
Loss of libido
Disturbed sleep – early wakening
Loss of weight
Inability to relax

Source: Royal College of General Practitioners and Royal College of Psychiatrists (1993) *Psychiatry and General Practice*. London, Royal College of Psychiatrists. In press. Reproduced with permission.

Two symptoms are particularly important in diagnosis because they are relatively specific. Depressed patients lose the ability to enjoy anything (anhedonia) and experience a severe impairment of concentration. Another helpful distinguishing feature is the length of time symptoms have been present. The longer the symptoms have been present, especially if present every day, the more likely it is that the patient has a depressive illness rather than simple low spirits. A man who weeps in the consulting room is almost certainly depressed.

Algorithms and mnemonics

Clinical algorithms (flow-charts) provide a stepwise procedure for making decisions about diagnosis and treatment of a clinical problem (Figure 1). They can supple-

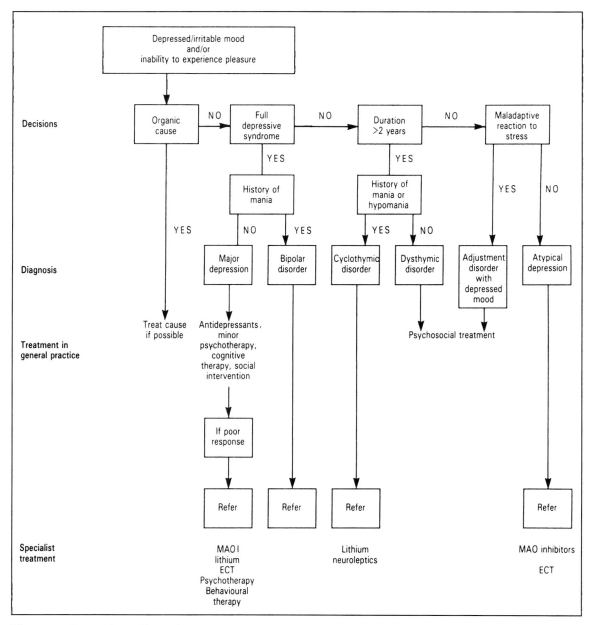

Figure 1 *Depression – diagnosis and treatment.*
Adapted from: Bhatera V (1984) The treatment of depression in primary care: decision-making aided by an algorithm. *South Dakota Journal of Medicine* **37**, 5–9.

ment, but do not replace, clinical judgement. They can also help the doctor develop a rational approach to the everyday problems of managing psychiatric illness in general practice.

The DSM III lists the signs and symptoms of

major depressive disorder (Table 3) and this definition is now widely accepted.

It can also be useful to have an *aide-mémoire* of the main features of depressive illness and this is provided by the mnemonic IN SAD CAGES (Rund and Hutzler, 1983; Table 5).

Table 5 *Mnemonic for depressive illness*

IN	**Interest** lost in nearly all activities because of inability to obtain pleasure from them.
S	**Sleep** disturbance and early morning wakening, at least two hours before the normal time.
A	**Appetite** is lost and weight loss (1 lb/wk) is common.
D	**Dysphoric** mood.
C	**Concentration** problems.
A	**Affect** blunted.
G	**Guilt** which is excessive, inappropriate and may be delusional.
E	**Energy** is lost. Inhibition of thought and drive.
S	**Suicidal ideation**.

Source: Rund and Hutzler (1983).

Psychiatric tests

Psychiatrists have experimented with various methods of defining and identifying depressive illness. There is even an experimental biochemical test for depression, the dexamethasone suppression test, but at present results are unreliable and it is of no practical value to general practitioners. Much useful work has been done using screening questionnaires (Hamilton, 1960; Goldberg, 1978), usually completed by the patient, followed by a structured interview by the psychiatrist to confirm the diagnosis (Goldberg et al., 1970; Montgomery and Asberg, 1979; Dean et al., 1983).

Patient-completed questionnaires are suitable for all but the very disturbed patient who may have difficulty in completing them but the answers depend to some extent on the patient's interpretation of the wording used. For example, the General Health Questionnaire (GHQ) is a self-reporting screening questionnaire which identifies individuals who have a high probability of suffering from psychological illness (Goldberg, 1972, 1978). The GHQ does not give a diagnosis but, especially when the depressed patient presents somatic symptoms or when depression is mixed with physical illness, it is useful in identifying hidden psychiatric illness (Goldberg and Blackwell, 1970; Tarnopolsky et al., 1979) and serves as a 'psychiatric ESR'.

Using this test in my own practice, I have been surprised how acceptable the GHQ is to patients and also, studying their answers, how successfully patients manage to continue their normal lives in the face of considerable misery and very distressing psychological symptoms (Wright and Perini, 1987). Another test which is useful clinically is the Hospital Anxiety and Depression questionnaire (Zigmond and Snaith, 1983), which provides separate scores for anxiety and depressive symptoms.

Modified versions of the stuctured psychiatric interviews can be of value in clinical practice as checklists of patient symptoms which change relatively quickly in response to therapy. For example, the Montgomery Asberg Depression Rating Scale (MADRS), lists 10 items which give a sensitive and accurate estimate of *change* in the patient's condition and can be helpful in following the progress of treatment (Montgomery and Asberg, 1979):

- apparent sadness
- reported sadness
- inner tension
- reduced sleep
- reduced appetite
- concentration difficulty
- lassitude
- inability to feel
- pessimistic thoughts
- suicidal thoughts.

Such tests can also help to distinguish transient disturbances of mood from depressive illness and to separate acute anxiety states from depression, which is not always easy in clinical practice. Depression can be missed if the doctor is too impressed by the patient's anxiety symptoms and the patient may be made worse by inappropriate prescribing of benzodiazepines, which often confuse the picture of developing depression and can also increase the risk of suicide.

Computer methods

In the last two decades computer interview systems have been developed in psychiatry and in some other fields (Dove et al., 1977). The computer program can ask as many questions as the doctor wishes and give patients as much time as they like to answer. Patients are truthful and accurate with the computer (Lucas, 1977) and in some cases the computer interview is a therapeutic experience for the patient and can improve the subsequent doctor/patient interview. Poyser (1985) advocates the use of the computer as a diagnostic tool in present day general practice. Experience in general practice shows that computer-based psychiatric testing is very acceptable to patients but that good organization and some extra staff time is required for their use within the confines of a normal working day (Wright, 1990). Tests which measure factors such as patient personality and socio-economic circumstances can be used in the same way.

While these tests can be educative to use and increase the doctor's awareness of patients' symptoms, they do not take the place of clinical judgement. One should not under-estimate the value of experience and clinical instinct and the ability to react to clues without necessarily understanding them fully. For example, general practitioners seem to be better than psychiatrists at picking up 'something' in patients who did not satisfy the criteria for depressive illness but were more likely to *become* depressed (MacDonald, 1986).

Widmer and Cadoret (1978) studied patient behaviour while they were developing their depressive illness just prior to diagnosis. They showed a significant increase in patient-initiated contacts in the 7-month period prior to diagnosis and it may be that this can be sensed by the general practitioner if not actually measured. It is also common for relatives of distressed patients to recognize depressive illness on the basis of changed behaviour. This is particularly true of patients who suffer from recurrent depressions whose relatives have seen these premonitory changes before and recognize their significance.

Missing psychiatric illness

General practitioners diagnose and manage a large number of depressed patients, referring less than 10% of those with recognized depression to secondary care services. However, many consulting patients who have depression are not recognized, especially when they complain mainly of physical symptoms. Patients known to the doctor as having true chronic physical illness are especially likely to be missed.

There is no shortage of evidence that many of these patients with significant psychiatric illness attending their general practitioner go unrecognized and untreated. Goldberg and Blackwell (1970) coined the term 'hidden psychiatric morbidity' and found that these patients were distinguished by their attitude to their illness and because they usually presented a physical problem to their doctor. Skuse and Williams (1984) studied psychiatric illness in a consecutive series of patients attending an experienced south London general practitioner. While the general practitioner diagnosed 24% of patients as having psychiatric illness, the true prevalence found by standardized psychiatric interview was 34%. The main reason for the difference was that the general practitioner gave a physical diagnosis to patients classified as depressed by psychiatric interview.

The reasons for non-diagnosis by general practitioners have been studied intensively (Marks et al., 1979; Goldberg et al., 1982; Davenport et al., 1987; Goldberg and Bridges, 1987) and it is clear that there are factors both within the doctor and the patient which make the detection of emotional disturbance less likely.

Reasons for non-diagnosis of depression

Patient factors

The most important of these is the tendency of some patients to somatize their psychological distress. Some patients consistently start the consultation by complaining of a physical symptom even though it is apparent that the main problem is psychological. This factor is particularly important in depressed patients as such patients have low self-esteem as part of the illness. Many are ashamed of their inability to cope with daily life and fear that the doctor will not take their complaints seriously. Some do not themselves recognize their distress as an illness and may present only the physical symptoms of their condition. This somatization is common but particularly so among ethnic minorities in the UK probably due partly to cultural factors and partly to difficulties with vocabulary and language.

Doctor factors

These include both bias of the doctor towards physical explanations for patient symptoms and his accuracy in diagnosing depression depending on his clinical experience. Doctors will miss vital non-verbal clues if they are looking at the notes rather than at the patient. Patients often give verbal clues of emotional distress when the doctor is concentrating on the physical examination. This is particularly so if the preliminaries have been hurried through by the doctor. Lastly, doctors commonly ask open questions about physical symptoms but are much less likely to offer an open question on emotional symptoms to the patient.

Nature of care system

In general practice this is radically different from the hospital system. Short appointments mean that primary complaints must be pursued at the expense of secondary and tertiary problems and that the diagnostic decision is normally spread over several consultations. This reason should not, however, be made an excuse. Longer consultations are often needed to deal adequately with the patient's emotional problem and the time must occasionally be found even if other patients are kept waiting. Often, a longer appointment can be arranged at a more suitable time to the doctor after initial assessment and negotiation with the patient

Improving recognition of depression

Although patient factors are important, better diagnosis depends largely on the clinical vigilance of the general practitioner. Most depressions which remain undiagnosed are 'missed' rather than 'masked' in the sense that the typical symptoms are present but the right questions are not asked.

The daily work of the general practitioner involves the responsibility to distinguish potentially life-threatening physical illness while managing very many and varied minor physical and social problems. These problems present unsorted to the consulting room and must be managed in a comparatively short consultation so that the doctor must move quickly from a fractious baby, to a sports injury, to a dermatological problem and then perhaps to a depressed patient who hurriedly offers only the physical symptoms of his complaint. Even with the best will and intentions on the part of the doctor, some depressed patients cannot be quickly diagnosed with confidence but will require several consultations for the correct diagnosis to emerge.

Ten-minute therapeutic consultation

While general practitioners do not normally have time for a full diagnostic interview, the normal 10-minute consultation can be used with advantage and can be effective both for recognition and for management. More time for the consultation would be welcomed both by doctor and patient but the important factor is not more time with the patient but a better use of the time already available. Time is not only spent in diagnosing depression but in negotiating with the patient what is to be done about the illness. Another important factor is continuity of care so the practice organization should help the patient to have appointments to be seen by the same doctor for the duration of the illness.

A good consulting style

Some doctors can recognize depression more easily than others (Lesser, 1985; Gask et al., 1987; Gask et al., 1988). Such doctors are usually 'good listeners', looking at the patient rather than the case notes and being less likely to interrupt the patient's story. Often such doctors have a special interest in psychiatry and are more knowledgeable about depression. They are usually directive in their consulting style but accept and make use of silence, using the patient's own answers to prompt further discussion.

Research has shown that case recognition can be improved by extra tuition in interviewing skills and a good consulting style can be developed by suitable training and practice (Goldberg et al., 1980). Using video feedback techniques, Gask et al. (1988) have demonstrated that interviewing skills can be improved and maintained over time. They have also shown that general practitioner trainers can be helped to pass on the skills to their own trainees (Gask et al., 1987). Criteria for a good interview style are given in Table 6.

Table 6 *Good interview style*

Begin with:
  Good eye contact
  Presenting symptom clearly established
  Directive questions for physical complaints
  Proceed from 'open' to 'closed' questions

Continue with:
  Emphatic style
  Sensitivity to verbal and *non-verbal* clues
  Avoid reading notes in front of patient
  Cope well with overtalkativeness

Screening and case finding

Screening for depression using questionnaires or computer-administered interviews has been shown to improve recognition under research conditions (Johnstone and Goldberg, 1976). Instruments can be used to identify probable psychiatric cases but these tests cannot make a clinical diagnosis. Screening can be useful clinically in raising the doctor's awareness of the possibility of depression and it is known that recognition improves outcome even when the patient does not comply with treatment (Freeling et al., 1985). Screening may be useful in high risk groups especially when the doctor is skilled and prepared to discuss social and psychological problems with the patient.

Masked depression and somatization

One of the most difficult problems the general practitioner faces in diagnosis is the patient who *persistently* presents with somatic complaints in the absence of any sign of physical abnormality. It is now recognized that many patients with depressive illness present physical symptoms to the doctor and may not volunteer any psychiatric symptoms and that depression can occur without any clear evidence of dysphoria (Remi et al., 1980; Bridges and Goldberg, 1985). Widmer and Cadoret (1978) showed that 26% of their series of depressed patients had somatic symptoms but that only 9% had purely physical complaints. Thus only a minority of patients showed a pure psychiatric presentation, while the majority had a mix of physical and psychological symptoms. These physical symptoms may be vegetative symptoms of depressive disorder or be part of the depressive 'vocabulary' of patients who normally somatize their psychological symptoms. The distress of chronic physical disease may also be made worse by the development of a depressive illness.

This phenomenon of presenting physical symptoms to the doctor and not the underlying psychological problem is referred to as somatization, which can be defined formally as "an idiom of distress in which patients with psychological and emotional problems articulate their distress primarily through physical symptomatology" (Katon et al., 1981). The concept of somatization is now widely recognized (Grol, 1988) but, of course, depression can also be 'missed' rather than 'masked' if the doctor does not think to ask the right questions.

Depression may have many 'masks' which vary according to age, education and ethnic background. The commonest presenting symptoms of masked depression are headache and excessive tiredness or weakness. Patients may also complain of lassitude, loss of energy, sleep disturbance, appetite and weight changes, loss of sexual drive, multiple aches and pains, constipation, dizziness and chest pains.

Warning situations include the inexplicable worsening of pre-existing physical illness or the chronic complainer especially where there is switching between different body systems. The latter type of patient often has 'fat file' case notes containing many letters from different hospital departments explaining what is not wrong with the patient. These patients present with physical symptoms and act in a less depressed way, causing difficulties for the doctor not because the features of depression are absent but because key symptoms are hidden by a great deal of somatic 'interference'. These patients may prefer to consider themselves as under strain rather than as depressed: the doctor may need to *negotiate* the diagnosis of depression. It is important to be aware of these indirect presentations of depressive illness and to realize that treatment can be more difficult owing to the patient's lack of insight.

It is often difficult for the doctor to recognize these patients in the short time available for a single consultation. Unrecognized patients tend to have had their symptoms longer and they are just as depressed as those who are easily recognized (Freeling et al., 1985).

Patients who somatize

In managing these patients the doctor may need to *negotiate* the diagnosis of depression. Patients may know that they are miserable but not that there is an affective illness. They may wish to negotiate in physical terms in spite of the psychological distress which is the main feature of the illness. This type of patient may prefer to think of himself as under strain rather than as depressed. Depressive illness diminishes the ability to cope with normal life situations. These 'somatization' symptoms may be a defence which protects the patient from psychological pain.

These patients respond to the same treatments as other people with depression but both the diagnosis and treatment must be negotiated with the patient rather than simply diagnosing depression and prescribing antidepressants. It is important to take a *full* history and to do a physical examination appropriate to the symptoms of which the patient is complaining. The patient should be made to feel that his or her distress is understood by the doctor, who can then probe his or her mood state while exploring social and family factors. The doctor should show empathy, recognizing the reality of the patient's pain and trying to understand his or her health beliefs. The patient who feels understood will come to accept the link between physical symptoms and the depressed mood, realizing that being depressed may lower resistance to 'normal' pains. The doctor may demonstrate that anxiety can cause muscle tension, which can cause pain. Sometimes symptoms such as non-organic headache may be common in a family, allowing the doctor to explain shared family behaviours.

5

Managing depression in general practice

GENERAL practitioners are well placed to help their depressed patients, who may have social problems and physical illness to cope with in addition to their depression. Treatment at home is usually best for the patient who is able to maintain ties with family and friends and may even be able to continue at work. Day unit care is useful for the more severe cases especially where there is little support from family or friends or where there is need for extended rehabilitation. Most depressed patients are treated entirely within primary care and even relatively severe depression can be treated in the community if the suicide risk is judged to be low and if the doctor is prepared to devote adequate time for the task, being willing to follow up patients appropriately throughout the whole course of the illness.

General assessment

Before deciding on management for an individual patient an individual assessment is needed. The patient must not only be given a diagnosis of depression but must also be assessed in physical, social and personality terms; and assessment must be made of psychosocial stresses and the effectiveness of support from family and friends. It is important to talk also about life events: patients with depression have more commonly experienced distressing life events such as bereavement, job loss or marriage breakdown in the six months prior to presentation. Systematic counselling should be deferred until after symptoms have improved and the patient is more able to respond.

A series of short appointments should be offered as this gives the opportunity to explore the history and symptoms in a systematic way without being too disruptive of ordinary consulting sessions. Frequent short appointments are not only very supportive for patients but regular attendance is valuable in ensuring proper compliance with drug regimes and other therapies. It is often not possible to analyse or to deal adequately with a psychological problem at the first presentation and many general practitioners prefer to make a special long appointment for problem patients or those who present diagnostic difficulty. It is useful to have a standard method for assessing psychiatric state for all patients who show disturbed behaviour or complain of emotional problems:

- Psychiatric status
- Suicide risk
- Personality characteristics
- Family history
- Social situation – stresses and supports
- Level of intelligence/ability to comply with treatment
- Physical morbidity.

A general psychiatric assessment devised by Rankin (1984) is listed in Table 7.

Assessing the risk of suicide

Assessing the risk of suicide is essential in all cases and patients should be referred promptly if a serious risk is present. Occasional thoughts about suicide are not in themselves cause for alarm as they are almost universal in severe depression. Important warnings are preoccupation with thoughts of suicide, active plans

Table 7 *General psychiatric assessment*

1. **Appearance and behaviour**
   This involves a thumbnail sketch of the patient's current status and behaviour.

2. **Speech**
   Speech should be noted for form, speed, coherence and absence of logical order.

3. **Mood**
   It is important to describe the patient's mood in the words he uses himself rather than in medical jargon. The patient should always be asked about suicidal thoughts or plans.

4. **Thought content**
   Ask if the patient has any special worries or preoccupations.

5. **Abnormal beliefs**
   It may be appropriate to ask specifically if the patient feels he is being watched, plotted against, or being influenced by others.

6. **Abnormal experiences**
   This includes hallucinations and other perceptual phenomena.

7. **Cognitive status**
   Check the patient's orientation in time and place and estimate intelligence and concentration. Brief tests of cognitive function are available such as the Mini Mental State Examination.

8. **Insight**
   Mental illness need not involve loss of insight and the patient may be asked whether he thinks he is ill or not and whether he regards his illness as physical or not.

and the fear that the urge might prove irresistible.

It is best to have open discussion of suicide in all patients in whom suicide is a reasonable possibility: most severely distressed patients are grateful to have the subject explored tactfully. There is no evidence that discussion can suggest ideas of suicide to the patient. It is best to work up from relatively gentle questions otherwise denial may be too ready. A series of suitable questions is, as follows:

- "Does it sometimes feel so bad that you feel you cannot take any more?"

- "Do you ever feel that it is just not worth going on?"

- "Have you ever thought about doing anything about it yourself?"

- "What had you thought of doing?"

- "What do you think stopped you from carrying it through?"

- "Would that work if you felt like that again?"

The doctor must try to distinguish serious suicide risk from suicidal gestures common especially in some female patients with personality disorders. The question "Have you ever wished you could simply go to sleep and not wake up again?" can give an early indication of suicidal impulse as it estimates the patient's subconscious wish to remove himself from his current stresses.

Suicide risk factors

Much background information will already be known to the general practitioner who must remember to use it. Risk factors include:

- Intense feelings of hopelessness and worthlessness

- Depression with marked sleep disturbance

- Poor physical health or much pain

- Living alone

- Recent stress or loss

- Male patient especially if over 45 years

- Alcoholism or heavy drinking

- Previous psychiatric illness or suicide attempt

- Family history of mental illness or suicide

- Family history of alcoholism.

Special risk factors in women

Special risk factors in women have been identified in a large survey by Brown and Harris (1978):

- Loss of mother by death or separation before age 12
- Three or more children under age 5
- Lack of either a close, caring relationship or a job.

Compulsory admission

Compulsory admission is rarely necessary in general practice. However, one should remember that most psychiatrists will admit a number of suicidally depressed patients under the Mental Health Act (Section 4) each year. For compulsory emergency admission an application by the nearest relative or an approved social worker is needed and the application must be supported by the opinion of a doctor.

The application must state:

1. That the patient is suffering from a mental disorder which warrants detention in a hospital for assessment.

2. That the patient ought to be detained in the interests of his/her own health or safety or to protect other persons.

3. That admission is urgent and the usual procedure would involve undesirable delay.

Treatment possibilities

A very important factor in improving outcome is simply recognition by the doctor and acceptance by the patient that he or she is suffering from an illness and that the prospects for cure are excellent. Simple reassurance and support and offering frequent short appointments is important for all patients but is not enough, and patients should not be denied the relief of antidepressant drugs or referral where appropriate. More could be probably be achieved within the existing system by making greater use of supportive therapies but one must first define the aims of the therapies and who can be helped.

Depressed patients are an important group because of their numbers, because their need is greater, and because they are less likely to be helped by social measures. All treatment possibilities may not be available to every practice. They are:

- Medication
- Supportive psychotherapy (doctor or community psychiatric nurse)
- Behaviour therapy (eg relaxation techniques, tapes)
- Cognitive therapy (understanding mental mechanisms which lead to depression)
- Social intervention (if remedial)
- Referral.

Antidepressant medication

Although drug therapy should not be the doctor's only response to depressive illness, antidepressant drugs have a crucial role in relieving the misery of a great many patients suffering from this painful illness. Antidepressants are used to relieve suffering, to shorten an episode of depression and sometimes to maintain against relapse.

It is fashionable to undervalue antidepressants and to overestimate the role of support/counselling – especially so when there has been much media publicity on benzodiazepine dependence increasing patient suspicion of any drug therapy. Current theories associate depressive illness with a deficiency in monoamines in certain areas of the brain and antidepressants may work by correcting this deficiency. Whether this is so or not it is a useful concept to explain therapy and encourage compliance particularly in patients who are reluctant to take any drugs or who are worried about becoming drug dependent. These patients may accept the idea of a temporary deficiency disease requiring replacement, for example diabetics who need insulin replacement.

The range of activity of antidepressants is wide and they are likely to be effective in most general practice patients given a diagnosis of depression or anxiety/depression. Antidepressants should be used where the syndrome of depression can be diagnosed (Paykel et al., 1992) and not withheld solely because the depression appears to be reactive to stressful life events or because the depression is understandable to the doctor. Clinically significant depression, the depressive syndrome, can be diagnosed when, in addition to persistent depressed mood, there are features such as pessimistic thought, suicidal feelings, sleep and appetite disturbance, severe impairment of energy, interest or concentration, to the extent that the patient's capacity to cope with normal living is impaired.

Successful treatment depends on adequate dosage and duration of therapy. Research has shown that many patients referred to outpatient clinics as chronic cases have not received the minimum therapeutic dose of antidepressant (Tyrer, 1978).

Antidepressants have been shown to be superior to placebo and to be effective in general practice. A wide range of effective drugs is now offered for use in general practice though no single antidepressant has been shown to be clearly superior to others. Drug choice is often made on the basis of side-effects or other medical conditions (heart disease glaucoma, epilepsy or enlarged prostate). By no means all the antidepressants prescribed are actually taken by the patient. Sometimes drugs are taken in inadequate dosage or for insufficient time.

Antidepressants may be less acceptable to patients than benzodiazepines because they are slower to take effect (14 days) and may cause unpleasant anticholinergic side-effects. It is important not to concentrate too much on the the manifestations of anxiety in depressed patients or their family carers or the doctor may neglect the possibility of depression. In patients with mixed anxiety/depression diazepam is not superior to placebo whereas antidepressant is. Patients who appear to suffer dramatic side-effects from very small doses of standard antidepressants may not have true depressive disorder and often are of a histrionic disposition.

Tricyclic and related antidepressants

Tricyclic antidepressants are the drugs most commonly used for depression in general practice where they have been available for over thirty years. They are cheap, effective, relatively safe in long-term use and their side-effects are well known. Tricyclics can be divided roughly into drugs with additional sedative properties (for example, amitriptyline) and those that are less sedative (for example, imipramine). Improvement in sleep pattern is usually the earliest benefit from therapy but it usually takes two to four weeks for the full antidepressant action to develop.

It is most important to build up to adequate therapeutic doses to provide plasma drug levels for effective treatment (for example, amitriptyline 150–200 mg per day). A good rule of thumb is to keep the patient on the maximum dose he/she can tolerate without troublesome side-effects. Treatment should be continued for 3 months to a year or more. Several trials have demonstrated the efficacy of 6-month maintenance therapy in preventing relapse.

It is not recommended to use combinations of drugs of the tricyclic group as this may constitute a hazard and side-effects are not reduced (BMA and RPSGB, 1992). Likewise mixtures of tricyclics with tranquillizers are not recommended. Though anxiety is common in depressive illness and may be the most prominent presenting symptom, the prescribing of antipsychotics or tranquillizers is seldom appropriate and may mask the diagnosis of depression.

The half life of tricyclic antidepressants is relatively long and they need be given only once per day, though one can start at a low dose three times a day and build up to a single dose at bedtime to lessen daytime drowsiness. Lower starting doses are appropriate in elderly patients (say 30–50% of the normal dose) as they are particularly sensitive to the hypotensive effects of this group of drugs and may suffer dizziness or even syncope. Dosages should be increased gradually but it is just as important in the elderly to achieve adequate therapeutic doses. At the beginning of treatment it is helpful to measure blood pressure lying and standing as marked postural hypotension is a good indicator of probable side-effects as the dosage is increased.

Particular care is needed in patients with cardiac disease as arrhythmias or heart block occasionally follow the use of tricyclics, although these problems are very rarely seen in general practice. Tricyclics can interfere with the action of some older hypotensives such as bethanidine, clonidine and guanethidine but fortunately do not cause problems with beta-blockers. Drugs of this group should be used with caution in epileptics as they lower the convulsion threshold.

One should always remember that tricyclics are dangerous in overdosage. It is advisable to see patients frequently at the early stages to chart progress, assess the suicide risk, and to prescribe a limited quantity of tablets, thus reducing the likelihood of problems with deliberate overdosage. The risk of overdosage is less with the newer drugs like mianserin.

Trials done in community samples (Porter, 1970; Blashki et al., 1971; Hollyman et al., 1988) show that tricyclic antidepressants are effective in the patients with moderate to severe depression seen in general practice using standard doses used in psychiatric practice (125–150 mg daily). Research evidence is less clear on the effectiveness of doses of 75 mg daily or lower, although clinical experience suggests that a minority of patients seem to stay well on such doses and to relapse on withdrawal.

Normally the doctor would start with a small dose to minimize side-effects increasing the dose till therapeutic levels are achieved. This usually takes two to three weeks on full dosage. The patient should be reassured that the treatment is not addictive and warned of both the expected delay in response and the common side-effects. These can be explained as 'a sign that the medicine is working'. When prescribing tricyclics, care is required with the elderly and in those with epilepsy or diabetes. Anticholinergic effects can cause problems in patients with glaucoma or enlarged prostate. Tricyclics are contra-indicated in severe liver disease and, because of cardiotoxicity, in recent myocardial infarction or in heart block.

The older tricyclic drugs have the major disadvantage of high toxicity in overdose making them generally unsuitable for unsupervised use in patients where there is risk of suicide attempt by overdosage.

The main side-effects of the tricyclic group are:

- Sedation (except imipramine)
- Postural hypotension
- Anticholinergic effects, for example dry mouth, constipation, urinary retention and blurred vision
- Weight gain, especially in middle-aged plump females.

Occasionally the general practitioner may settle for prescribing a lower dose antidepressant for its effect on sleep and this is often acceptable to patients. Patient attitudes affect compliance especially when there are significant social stress factors as the patient does not easily accept that these are likely to be helped by drugs. Media coverage of benzodiazepine dependence makes patients less likely to accept medication. A patient may find antidepressants more acceptable if he believes that sleep benefits or lowered anxiety will enable him to make better use of his own resources.

In middle-aged over-weight women the most troublesome side-effect of all is marked increase in weight due to therapy. These patients are, understandably, particularly reluctant to continue maintenance therapy once their symptoms have been relieved.

This problem does not seem to occur with trazodone, which is the drug of choice in these circumstances.

Prescribing for special groups

For young people with no complicating factors many doctors will prefer to use the well tried, tested and relatively safe amitriptyline when sedation is also desired. If the patient is withdrawn or apathetic imipramine may be prescribed for its activating effect. Some of the newer drugs, for example lofepramine or fluvoxamine are less toxic on overdose. When the risk of suicide is high, electroconvulsive therapy is often preferable.

Old people have less efficient metabolism and excretion, which results in increased sensitivity to drugs. Older people are more likely to be on other drugs which might interact, for example hypotensives, antacids, or cimetidine. One must particularly beware of the hypotensive effects of tricyclics which can lead to giddiness and falls. Anticholinergic side-effects may precipitate urinary retention in men with enlarged prostates, constipation can go on to impaction, and glaucoma can cause blurred vision leading to injury. Dry mouth is unpleasant but, if it leads to polydipsia and excessive fluid intake, circulatory overload can ensue. For these reasons many doctors prefer, for their older patients, to use lofepramine, mianserin or dothiepin, which have fewer side-effects. In any case it is best to use 30–50% of normal adult dose and build up slowly looking for side-effects and seeing the patient regularly to prevent drug toxicity effects. Benzodiazepines should be avoided as they may exacerbate symptoms in a confused patient.

Dysthymia responds less well to antidepressants. Psychotherapy, including cognitive therapy, or relevant social intervention is likely to be more effective.

Selective serotonin reuptake inhibitors

The place of the newer antidepressant drugs, including the selective serotonin reuptake inhibitors (SSRI, also called 5HT antagon-ists), is still controversial (Matthews and Eagles, 1991), though they are significantly less toxic in overdose and their cleaner side-effect profile will probably make them more acceptable to patients. They have fewer effects on the cardiovascular system than the familiar tricyclics and fewer irksome anticholinergic effects. The main side-effects are gastro-intestinal with nausea being particularly troublesome in some patients.

The effectiveness of this group of drugs has been demonstrated by placebo-controlled trials but few trials have been carried out in elderly depressed patients. There is less information on long-term safety than is available on the older drugs. As they are new drugs with unknown teratogenic properties it would seem wise to avoid using them in pregnancy at present. SSRI drugs are at present much more expensive than the familiar tricyclic antidepressants. Edwards (1992) has recently classified the selective serotonin reuptake inhibitors as "a modest though welcome advance in the treatment of depression".

Other antidepressant drugs

Two other groups of drugs are also used to treat depressive illness, namely monoamine-oxidase inhibitors (MAOI) and lithium salts. Therapy by monoamine-oxidase inhibitors is often initiated by specialists because of the dangers of dietary and drug interactions which can cause a dangerous rise in blood pressure. Lithium salts are used in the treatment of bipolar disorder (manic depressive illness) and patients require regular blood sampling to control therapeutic levels.

Monoamine oxidase inhibitors

Monoamine oxidase inhibitors are normally reserved for patients who have not responded to other antidepressants or those with 'atypical depression' described in a previous chapter (2). Close supervision of these patients is required, especially regarding diet, to avoid precipitating hypertensive crises. Treatment is probably best initiated by a specialist who may also consider adding lithium to the drug regime.

Lithium salts

Lithium was first used by Cade (1949) in Australia to treat manic depressive illness. It is a valuable prophylactic and, properly used, it is much less toxic to the kidneys than was first thought. There are now indications for its use, with care, in general practice. Dosage is controlled by sampling blood levels.

Lithium is normally used, with major tranquillizers, in acute mania or hypomania and is effective within a few days. It is useful for long-term prophylaxis of depression in bipolar disorder and there may be some advantage in adding lithium to the antidepressant regime of some depressives who fail to respond to standard therapy. There is quite strong evidence from trials that lithium is of value in preventing relapse in recurring depression.

Appendix 1 lists the drugs commonly used to treat depression together with their basic NHS cost.

Maintenance therapy: preventing relapse

After symptoms have been relieved it is wise to continue treatment for several months and the question of preventing relapse should be considered and discussed with the patient. Research work has shown that inadequate therapy in the first six months of treatment results in relapse rates as high as 50% compared with 20% where treatment is continued. To prevent relapse, a further four to six months of treatment is recommended after symptoms have been relieved at the dose at which a clinical response was achieved. It can be difficult to persuade a newly well patient to continue prophylactic drug therapy for this length of time but such prophylaxis is well worthwhile.

Longer term prophylactic drug therapy extending beyond the first phase of six months is controversial and is still a matter for clinical judgement. Long-term lithium therapy is appropriate for manic-depressive illness and it is worthwhile considering continuing tricyclic antidepressants for recurring severe depression though there is neither consensus on appropriate dosage of antidepressants for long-term use nor on recommended total duration of prophylaxis. Available evidence suggests that it is necessary to continue relatively high doses to achieve effective prophylaxis. If longer term high dose treatment seems appropriate, the decision should be taken jointly with the patient after explaining risks and potential benefits.

6

Non-drug treatment

WHILE some patients do not wish to take drugs for their depression and others will not respond to drugs alone, the choice is not between drugs and other therapy but which combination of drugs and psychosocial treatment is most appropriate in the individual case. Most depressed people are helped by appropriate psychosocial approaches to management.

Formal counselling within the practice should be deferred until the acute distress has been relieved by antidepressant drugs. In the early stages any psychotherapy will be of a supportive type but as symptoms improve a more problem-oriented and intensive approach may be appropriate. Normally the general practitioners would identify the problems that the patient feels that he or she is facing and try to establish the patient's personal priorities. It is often worthwhile to seek the support of family and friends, self-help groups or support groups run by community psychiatric nurses or other health professionals. Discussing chronic social difficulties or relationship problems often brings relief to the patient even though he may feel powerless to change.

Other more specialized non-drug therapies may be considered with advantage but not all therapies will be available to the general practitioner. These special therapies can be useful in the type of depression found in general practice (Tyrer, 1988; Andrews, 1991). Cognitive therapy is a useful additional measure in treatment and prophylaxis and the skills can be learned by a general practitioner or community psychiatric nurse.

Cognitive therapy

Cognitive therapy aims to demonstrate to the patient that his pessimistic assumptions are based on illogical argument and are not justified by the facts. It can help the patient to understand the illness and the cause, where this can be traced to harmful patient behaviour or attitudes.

Depressed patients tend to think negatively rather than positively, tend to be pessimistic rather than optimistic, and to undervalue their own achievements. This can be counteracted to some extent by cognitive therapy which is also useful in rehabilitation of patients when the depression has passed. Simple help, support and common sense advice is often effective and attention to 'life-style management' may prevent further attacks.

Cognitive therapy can be effective and cost efficient with depressed patients in general practice (Teasdale et al., 1984; Ross and Scott, 1985). Patients whose depression has become chronic and those with major social stresses are those most likely to respond to this approach and benefits from this treatment are known to be maintained for at least a year. Psychology services vary considerably across the country and referrals should probably be restricted to resistant or recurrent problems.

Social intervention

This is probably less effective in depressive illness than in other forms of mental illness unless there are clear social problems involved in causation and unless these are remedial. Corney (1984) studied the effect of allocating patients a social worker for a 6-month period but was unable to show benefit. Much depends on patient motivation and the amount of practical help that can be given.

Counselling

Studies of brief counselling conducted by general practitioners have tended to be concerned with anxiety reduction techniques rather than the management of depressive illness. Depressed people with marital problems do well treated by counsellors attached to general practices. Women with postnatal depression have been shown to benefit from simple counselling by health visitors.

Voluntary organizations

Voluntary organizations can have a useful role in supporting the family carers and in assisting social readjustment after a long illness (Appendix 2). Some patients obtain benefit from attending local self-help groups.

Referral to a psychiatrist

The traditional view that the more severely depressed patients are all likely to be referred and managed by a consultant is true only of patients suffering from psychotic illness. Probably about 1 in 10 patients identified as having depressive illness are referred to psychiatrists. While many depressed patients are rightly referred for specialist help, referral of depressed patients is often made on the basis of additional complicating factors such as personality disorder, alcohol abuse, or family pressure for admission.

It is appropriate to refer whenever the general practitioner feels that guidance or help is required with diagnosis or management, for example when progress is unsatisfactory in spite of adequate treatment. When there is a high risk of suicide being attempted or when patients show markedly disturbed behaviour, particularly psycho-motor retardation, agitation, or psychotic features, they should be referred to a psychiatrist without delay.

Good communication between doctors is essential and must be two-way if the patient is to enjoy maximum benefit from the consultant's special skills.

A good referral letter

The psychiatrist likes to know what the general practitioner thinks of the problem and to have his local insights into possible precipitants of this illness. The general practitioner's knowledge of past history and family history is invaluable and must be communicated. Much time is saved if the psychiatrist knows *all* the drugs the patient is taking and their doses. It is helpful if he knows what drugs have been tried, at what doses, and for how long. Details of previous referral including the name of the psychiatrist consulted, the name of the hospital, and the patient's hospital number makes tracing of old records much easier.

A good reply

General practitioners appreciate, in the psychiatrist's letter of reply, some explanation of the decisions reached and the reasons for recommending a particular therapy. They also like to know what the patient has been told and what follow-up arrangements, if any, have been made. Good discharge letters can also have an important educational value. They should be addressed to the general practitioner and written primarily to meet his needs and not those of the hospital case notes (Yellowlees and Pullen, 1984).

Referral to a clinical psychologist

Psychologists can offer several measures including behaviour therapy, psychotherapy, and relaxation techniques often involving the use of individually prepared cassette tapes (Appendix 3).

Electroconvulsive therapy

Electroconvulsive therapy (ECT) is not used routinely in treating depression but, where the depressed patient shows psychotic features, there is risk from suicide, starvation or dehydration it can be life saving. The place of electroconvulsive therapy in treating severe depression is to some extent controversial and over exposure on the media has led to some suitable patients being denied the relief of this effective and remarkably safe therapy. ECT is the treatment of choice for suicidal depressives, for delusional depres-

sives and for recurrent depression which has previously responded well to this therapy. Severe depression with stupor is rarely seen, even by psychiatrists, but ECT is then strongly indicated.

Figure 2 gives a flow chart for the treatment of depression. A reading list giving details of books suitable for doctors and for patients is given in Appendix 4.

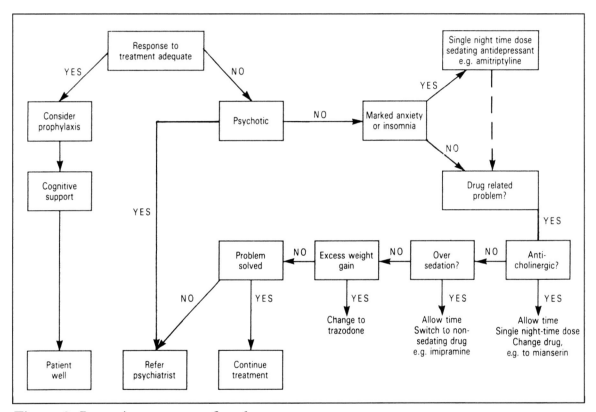

Figure 2 *Depression – treatment flow chart.*

Auditing and quality assurance

IT IS becoming common for primary care teams to develop protocols for the management of common chronic diseases in their practices and to monitor their compliance with these protocols through clinical audit. Teams now expect not only to look after patients but to define aims and test whether they are reaching their standards for the process and outcome of their clinical care. Such management protocols are common in the management of diabetes, asthma and hypertension but are rarely in place for the care of mental illness.

The care of depressive illness in general practice is a worthwhile area for performance review of both process and outcome. Checking that adequate doses of antidepressant are being prescribed for an adequate length of time would itself have a significant effect on treatment outcomes. Systematic performance review of patient follow-up would provide valuable information, especially on how successfully patients are being persuaded to comply with treatment.

Burton and Freeling (1982) have proposed a practical method of record keeping for the management of depression in a practice so that process of care can be reviewed reliably. Such clinical performance review has the potential for substantial benefits to the patient.

Prevention

ALTHOUGH there has been progress in the prevention of major physical illness this has not been matched in psychiatric illness in general or depression in particular. There is good evidence for continuing an antidepressant for six months after relief of symptoms and this should be standard practice. Long-term prophylactic therapy with antidepressants is probably justified in some patients with frequently recurring depression. The hope of 'behavioural immunization' for those suffering recurrent depression has been realized only in the small minority of patients in whom social or personality factors are clearly important in precipitating relapse or recurrence.

The personality of the patient has long been recognized as central to the successful management of most diseases in general practice and there is no doubt that in some vulnerable individuals personality attributes increase the likelihood of becoming depressed. It has also been shown in patients in general practice with psychiatric illness that there are measurable personality differences between those who present physical problems to the doctor and those who consult for psychological symptoms (Wright, 1990). In reality it is much easier to recognize personality differences than to measure them and the difficulty of assessing personality in the presence of depression must be remembered. It was formerly believed that obsessional personalities had a tendency to have 'endogenous' type symptoms while 'neurotic' symptoms were linked to those with neurotic personality traits. This distinction proved of little value in clinical practice.

It is reasonable to suppose that patients facing life stresses would be more vulnerable to depressive illness and recent work supports this view. Vulnerability factors include the absence of a confiding relationship, unemployment, caring for young children and the loss of a mother in childhood. In family practice it is obvious that a confiding relationship with spouse, family or close friend is of great benefit both in treating and trying to prevent recurrence. Similarly, contact with a sympathetic social worker is helpful when social problems are remedial.

Depressed patients can be helped to reverse their negative attitude of themselves and to be convinced that anxiety-producing situations at work or in social contacts can be controlled and need not cause their depression to return.

Managing 'difficult' patients

SOME patients are notoriously difficult to please, repeatedly presenting their general practitioner with a wide and varying range of symptoms, mostly somatic. There is often no precise psychiatric diagnosis possible and they may be thought of as being hypochondriacal or histrionic or as having a minor personality disorder. Some of these patients may be depressed and may respond to a proper trial of antidepressants in adequate dose if they can be persuaded to persist with treatment. Most will continue to follow the same behaviour patterns but benzodiazepines should not be prescribed as they create more problems than they solve. A gentle supportive relationship with the doctor is probably the best management, though it may be necessary to have a 'contract' with the patient to see him or her only at regular scheduled times, as such patients can be very stressful for the doctor to deal with. Many of these patients have poor interpersonal relationships because of their antisocial behaviour. They may be prone to outbursts of anger, causing problems for the receptionist staff.

Depression and physical disease

PHYSICAL and psychological illness frequently co-exist and certain individuals are particularly prone to both types of illness. This connection between the physical and the psychological has been recognized for many centuries in the term melancholia, a condition of mind and body traditionally attributed to an 'excess of the black bile'.

Chronic painful, disfiguring or incapacitating illness can very understandably lead to low spirits and depressed mood. Certain patients seem to be especially susceptible to both physical and psychological illness and patients who are very dependent on others for care seem more likely to become depressed. Some illnesses are particularly associated with depressive disorder, for example cancer, Crohn's disease, diabetes, and other endocrine and metabolic diseases. Painful bone disorders and neurological disease, especially multiple sclerosis, are strongly linked to depressive illness. Depression associated with these physical illnesses carries a high risk of suicide but fortunately it does respond to antidepressant drugs.

Sudden cataclysmic physical events (infarct, coronary artery bypass, stroke) can be followed by a severe depressive reaction, perhaps owing to the psychological trauma of facing death. In these circumstances vigorous treatment of the depressive reaction can take precedence over the management of the physical disease, for example a patient with advanced cancer of the lung who becomes severely depressed.

Somatization

Patients with co-existing physical illness are particularly likely to conceal their depression by somatization, either causing an exacerbation of their existing physical disease or producing new physical symptoms. Unless the depression is recognized and treated, full recovery from the organic disease may be delayed or prevented. Depression in these patients may not present in the usual textbook manner and the other manifestations of the physical illness further confuse the clinical picture.

Working together

IN several ways psychiatrists have more in common with general practitioners than have most specialists. Both are particularly interested in treating the whole patient in his environment and both are less dependent than most specialists on high technology. Up to 25% of patients consult their family doctor for problems which are wholly or partly psychological. With the rapid reduction in institutional care many more patients with chronic psychoses or learning disabilities are living in the community and seeking care from general practitioners. These movements have led to more psychiatrists working in the community with various models of shared care being developed, including psychiatrists consulting in health centres in contact with the practice team, other health professionals, and social workers (Mitchell, 1984). This arrangement has been especially popular in Scotland (Strathdee and Williams, 1984). As a result of these changes in the traditional working relationships between primary and secondary care a working group was set up between the Royal Colleges of General Practitioners and Psychiatrists (1993) to examine the most appropriate models of shared care between the specialties.

Meaningful communication is particularly important between general practitioner and psychiatrist but letters are not always satisfactory (Yellowlees and Pullen, 1984), and using the telephone can be time wasting. There are distinct advantages in specialist consultation for the patient in a health centre or general practice surgery: the patient is spared the ordeal of attending a hospital psychiatric clinic and communication between psychiatrist and general practitioner is greatly enhanced. Both general practitioners and specialists find these liaison arrangements satisfactory (Strathdee, 1988).

Personal experience of one model of liaison in my own health centre has convinced me of its benefit to specialist, general practice team and patient. Personal contact leads to more consistent and co-ordinated treatment while discussion with the psychiatrist helps uncover the 'hidden agenda' of the general practitioner's problem with his patient's management that is often difficult to detail adequately in a letter. Good liaison simplifies treatment policies, for example for drug or alcohol abusers, improves the selection of patients referred, and establishes a consensus on handing back referred patients.

The visiting psychiatrist can reinforce the confidence of the primary care team in its ability to manage psychiatric problems wholly in the community. He has a central role in helping general practitioners to refine management and audit skills as well as improving detection.

Conclusion

DEPRESSION is a very common illness in general practice and causes much distress and under-achievement. It is not a mild, self-limiting disease and, despite advances in knowledge, it is still under-diagnosed and under-treated to an important extent. Some patients do not approach their doctor directly with psychological symptoms and some do not seek treatment at all because of the perceived stigma of mental illness. The Royal College of Psychiatrists and the Royal College of General Practitioners have co-operated in a joint initiative on depression which aims to make doctors and other health professionals more aware of the disease and convince the public that depression is an illness and not a lack of moral fibre.

Depression is a major challenge for the primary health care team. It is an eminently treatable disease with a high probability of cure and enhancement of the quality of patients' lives. It should be actively looked for, carefully supervised and energetically treated. It can be very satisfying for the doctor to manage and few patients are more grateful to their doctor than those successfully treated for depressive illness.

Acknowledgement

I am grateful to Dr Michael King, Senior Lecturer and Consultant Psychiatrist at the Royal Free Hospital, London for constructive criticism of the typescript. For the diary of a depressed patient (Appendix 5) and for advising on relaxation techniques (Appendix 3) I am indebted to Dr AS Presley, Principal Clinical Psychologist, Stratheden Hospital, Fife.

References

American Psychiatric Association (1987) Diagnostic and Statistical Manual of Mental Disorders (3rd ed. revised). Washington, APA.

Andrews G (1991) The evaluation of psychotherapy. *Current Opinion in Psychiatry* **4**, 379-83.

Anonymous (1989) A GP trainee's personal story of depression. *RCGP Connection.* London, RCGP. pp 2-3.

Balint M (1964) *The Doctor, His Patient and the Illness.* 2nd ed. London, Pitman.

Barber J H (1981) Depressive illness in general practice. *Acta Psychiatrica Scandinavica* (suppl.) 414-46.

Blashki TG, Mowbray R and Davies B (1971) Controlled trial of amitriptyline in general practice. *British Medical Journal* **1**, 133-8.

Blacker CVR and Clare AW (1987) Depressive disorder in primary care. *British Journal of Psychiatry* **150**, 737-51.

Bridges K and Golberg DP (1985) Somatic presentations of DSM-III psychiatric disorders in primary care. *Journal of Psychosomatic Research* **29**, 563-9.

British Medical Association and Royal Pharmaceutical Society of Great Britain (1992) *British National Formulary.* London, BMA and Pharmaceutical Press.

Brown GW and Harris T (1978) *Social Origins of Depression: A Study of Psychiatric Disorder in Women.* London, Tavistock Publications.

Buchan IC and Richardson IM (1973) *Time Study of Consultations in General Practice. Scottish Health Services Studies No. 27.* Edinburgh, Scottish Home and Health Department.

Burton RH and Freeling P (1982) How general practitioners manage depressive illness: developing a method of audit. *Journal of the Royal College of General Practitioners* **33**, 558-61.

Cade JFJ (1949) Lithium salts in the treatment of psychotic excitement. *Medical Journal of Australia* **2**, 349-52.

Casey PR (1990) *A Guide To Psychiatry in Primary Care.* Petersfield, Wrightson.

Casey PR, Dillon S and Tyrer PJ (1984) The diagnostic status of patients with conspicuous psychiatric morbidity in primary care. *Psychological Medicine* **14**, 673-83.

Chisholm J (1990) The Read clinical classification. *British Medical Journal* **300**, 1092.

Corney RH (1984) The effectiveness of attached social workers in the management of depressed female patients in general practice. *Psychological Medicine*, Suppl 6.

Croft-Jeffries C and Wilkinson G (1989) Costs of neurotic illness in UK general practice in 1985. *Psychological Medicine,* **19**, 549-58.

Davenport S, Goldberg D and Millar T (1987) How psychiatric disorders are missed during medical consultations. *Lancet* **1**, 439-41.

Dean C, Surtees PG and Sashidharan SP (1983) Comparisons of research diagnostic systems in an Edinburgh community sample. *British Journal of Psychiatry* **142,** 247-56.

Dove GAW, Wigg P, Clarke JHE et al. (1977) The therapeutic effect of taking a patient's history by computer. *Journal of the Royal College of General Practitioners* **27,** 477-81.

Dunn G and Skuse D (1981) The natural history of depression in general practice: stochastic models. *Psychological Medicine* **11**, 755-64.

Edwards JG (1992) Selective serotonin reuptake inhibitors. *British Medical Journal* **304,** 1644-5.

Freeling P, Rao BM, Paykel ES et al. (1985) Unrecognised depression in general practice. *British Medical Journal* **290,** 1880-3.

Gask L, Goldberg D, Lesser AL et al. (1988) Improving the psychiatric skills of the general practice trainee: an evaluation of a group training course. *Medical Education* **22,** 132-8.

Gask L, McGrath G and Goldberg D (1987) Improving the psychiatric skills of established general practitioners; evaluation of group teaching. *Medical Education* **21,** 362-8.

Goldberg DP (1972) *The Detection of Psychiatric Illness by Questionnaire.* London, Oxford University Press.

Goldberg DP (1978) *Manual of the General Health Questionnaire.* Slough, NFER-Wilson.

Goldberg DP (1985) Identifying psychiatric illness among general medical patients. *British Medical Journal* **291**, 161-2.

Goldberg DP (1986) Use of the General Health Questionnaire in clinical work. *British Medical Journal* **293,** 1188-9.

Goldberg DP and Blackwell B (1970) Psychiatric illness in general practice: a detailed study using a new method of case identification. *British Medical Journal* **2,** 439-43.

Goldberg D and Bridges K (1987) Screening for psychiatric illness in general practice: the general practitioner versus the screening questionnaire. *Journal of the Royal College of General Practitioners* **37**, 15-18.

Goldberg DP, Cooper B, Eastwood MR et al. (1970) A standard psychiatric interview for use in community surveys. *British Journal of Preventive and Social Medicine* **24**, 18-23.

Goldberg D and Huxley P (1992) *Common Mental Disorders: A Bio-Social Model.* London, Routledge.

Goldberg DP, Steele J, Smith C et al. (1980) Training family practice residents to recognise psychiatric disturbances. Final report to Dept. of Biometrics and Family Practice, Medical University of South Carolina.

Goldberg DP, Steele JJ, Johnson A et al. (1982) Ability of primary care physicians to make accurate ratings of psychiatric symptoms. *Archives of General Psychiatry* **39**, 829-33.

Grol R (1988) *To Heal or To Harm. The Prevention of Somatic Fixation in General Practice.* London, Royal College of General Practitioners.

Hamilton M (1960) A rating scale for depression. *Journal of Neurology, Neurosurgery and Psychiatry* **23**, 46-62.

Hoeper EW, Nyez GR, Cleary PD (1979) The Quality of Mental Health Services in an Organized Primary Care Setting. Final Report. Washington, National Institute of Mental Health.

Hollyman JA, Freeling P, Paykel ES et al. (1988) Double-blind placebo-controlled trial of amitriptyline among depressed patients in general practice. *Journal of the Royal College of General Practitioners* **38**, 393-7.

Jenkins R and Shepherd M (1983) Mental illness in general practice. In *Mental Illness: Changes and Trends.* Ed. Bean P. Chichester, Wiley.

Johnson DAW and Mellor V (1977) The severity of depression in patients treated in general practice. *Journal of the Royal College of General Practitioners* **27**, 419-22.

Johnstone A and Goldberg D (1976) Psychiatric screening in general practice: a controlled trial. *Lancet* **1**, 605-8.

Katon W, Kleinman A and Rosen G (1981) Depression and somatization: a review part 1. *American Journal of Medicine* **72**, 127-35.

Kendell RE (1975) *The Role of Diagnosis in Psychiatry.* London, Blackwells.

Kendell RE (1988) What is a case? *Archives of General Psychiatry* **45**, 374-6.

Lader M (1975) The social implications of psychotropic drugs. *Royal Society of Health Journal* **95b**, 304-5.

Lesser AL (1985) Problem-based interviewing in general practice: a model. *Medical Education* **19**, 299-304.

Lewis G, Pelosi AJ, Araya R et al. (1989) Measuring psychiatric disorder in the community: a standardized assessment for use by lay interviewers. *Psychological Medicine* **22**, 465-86.

Lucas RW (1977) A study of patients' attitudes to computer interrogation. *International Journal of Man-machine Studies* **9**, 69-86.

MacDonald AJD (1986) Do general practitioners 'miss' depression in elderly patients? *British Medical Journal* **292**, 1365-7.

Mann AH, Jenkins R and Belsey E (1981) The twelve month outcome of patients with neurotic illness in general practice. *Psychological Medicine* **11**, 535-50.

Marinker M (1973) The doctor's role in prescribing. In *The Medical Use of Psychotropic Drugs. Supplement No 2.* London, Journal of the Royal College of General Practitioners.

Marks J, Goldberg DP and Hillier VE (1979) Determinants of the ability of general practitioners to detect psychiatric illness. *Psychological Medicine* **9**, 337-53.

Matthews K and Eagles JM (1991) Which antidepressant? *British Journal of General Practice* **41**, 123-5.

Mitchell ARK (1984) A psychiatrist in the health centre. *Update* **15**, 1192-6.

Montgomery SA and Asberg M (1979) A new depression scale designed to be sensitive to change. *British Journal of Psychiatry* **134**, 382-9.

MORI Poll (1992) Attitudes towards Depression. Defeat Depression Campaign. For Royal College of Psychiatrists.

Overton GW and Wise TN (1980) Psychiatric diagnosis in family practice: is the General Health Questionnaire an effective screening instrument? *Southern Medical Journal* **73**, 763-4.

Paykel ES, Priest RG et al. (1992) Recognition and management of depression in general practice: consensus statement. *British Medical Journal* **305**, 1198-202.

Porter AMW (1970) Depressive illness in a general practice. A demographic study and a controlled trial of imipramine. *British Medical Journal* **1**, 773-8.

Poyser J (1985) Patient interviewing. In *Trends in General Practice Computing.* Ed. Sheldon M and Stoddart N. London, Royal College of General Practitioners. pp 176-82.

Rankin DW (1984) Psychiatric emergencies. *Medicine in Practice* **2**, 48-50.

Remi J, Cadoret MD, Reuben B et al. (1980) Depression in family practice: long-term prognosis and somatic complaints. *Journal of Family Practice* **10,** 625-9.

Robins LN, Helzer JE, Weissman MM et al. (1984) Lifetime prevalence of specific psychiatric disorders in three sites. *Archives of General Psychiatry* **41,** 949-58.

Ross M and Scott M (1985) An evaluation of the effectiveness of individual and group cognitive therapy in the treatment of depressed patients in the inner city health centre. *Journal of the Royal College of General Practitioners* **35,** 239-42.

Royal College of General Practitioners and Royal College of Psychiatrists (1993) Report of a working party on shared care. In preparation.

Rund DM and Hutzler J (1983) In Sad Cages: a mnemonic for depression. Letter. *American Journal of Psychiatry* **140,** 5.

Shepherd M, Cooper M, Brown AC et al. (1966) *Psychiatric Illness in General Practice.* (2nd ed. 1981) London, Oxford University Press.

Sims ACP and Salmons PH (1975) Severity of symptoms of psychiatric outpatients: use of the General Health Questionnaire in hospital and general practice patients. *Psychological Medicine* **5,** 62-6.

Skuse D and Williams P (1984) Screening for psychiatric disorder in general practice. *Psychological Medicine* **14,** 365-77.

Strathdee G (1988) Psychiatrists in primary care: the general practitioner's viewpoint. *Family Practice* **5,** 111-15.

Strathdee G and Williams P (1984) A survey of psychiatrists in primary care: the silent growth of a new service. *Journal of the Royal College of General Practititoners* **34,** 615-18.

Tarnopolsky A, Hand DJ, McLean EK et al. (1979) Validity and uses of a screening questionnaire (GHQ) in the community. *British Journal of Psychiatry* **134,** 508-15.

Teasdale JD, Fennell MJV, Hibbert GA et al. (1984) Cognitive therapy for major depressive disorders in primary care. *British Journal of Psychiatry* **144,** 400-6.

Thompson D and Pudney M (1990) *Mental Illness: The Fundamental Facts.* London, Mental Health Foundation.

Tyrer P (1978) Drug treatment of psychiatric patients in general practice. *British Medical Journal* **2,** 1008-10.

Tyrer P (1988) The Nottingham study of neurotic disorder: comparison of drug and psychological treatments. *Lancet* **2,** 235-40.

Widmer RB and Cadoret RJ (1978) Depression in primary care: changes in pattern of patient visits and complaints during a developing depression. *Journal of Family Practice* **7,** 293-302.

Widmer RB and Cadoret RJ (1979) Depression in family practice: changes in pattern of patient visits and complaints during subsequent developing depressions. *Journal of Family Practice* **9,** 1017-21.

Wilkin D and Williams EI (1986) Patterns of care for the elderly in general practice. *Journal of the Royal College of General Practitioners* **36,** 567-70.

Williams EI (1993) Mental health problems of old people. In *Psychiatry and General Practice.* London, Royal College of Psychiatrists. In press.

Williams EI and Wallace P (1993) *Health Checks for People Aged 75 and Over. Occasional Paper 59.* London, Royal College of General Practitioners. In press.

Williams P, Tarnopolsky A and Hand D (1980) Case definition and case identification in psychiatric epidemiology: review and assessment. *Psychological Medicine* **10,** 101-14.

Williamson J, Stokoe IH and Gray S (1964) Old people at home: the unreported needs. *Lancet* **1,** 1117-20.

World Health Organization (1978) *International Classification of Diseases.* 9th revision. Geneva, WHO.

Wright AF (1988) Psychological distress in a general practice: outcome and consultation rates. *Journal of the Royal College of General Practitioners* **38,** 542-5.

Wright AF (1990) A study of the presentation of somatic symptoms in general practice by patients with psychiatric disturbance. *British Journal of General Practice* **40,** 459-63.

Wright AF and Perini AF (1987) Hidden psychiatric illness: use of the General Health Questionnaire in general practice. *Journal of the Royal College of General Practitioners* **37,** 164-7.

Yellowlees AJ and Pullen IM (1984) Communication between psychiatrists and general practitioners. What sort of letters should psychiatrists write? *Health Bulletin* **42/6,** 285-96.

Zigmond A and Snaith RP (1983) The Hospital Anxiety and Depression Scale. *Acta Psychiatrica Scandinavica* **67,** 361-70.

The cost and dosage of antidepressant drugs

	Daily dose		Cost	
Sedative trycyclics	**Maintenance**	**Maximum**	**20 Tablets**	**30 Days**
Amitriptyline 25 mg	50–100 mg	150–200 mg	£0.08	£0.48
Lentizol cap 25 mg			£0.92	£5.52
Tryptizol tab 25 mg			£0.46	£2.76
Trimipramine 25 mg	75–150 mg	300 mg	★	★
Surmontil tab 25 mg			£1.65	£14.85
Dothiepin cap 25 mg	75 mg	150 mg	£0.95	£4.28
Prothiaden cap 25 mg			£1.00	£4.50
Mianserin 20 mg	30–90 mg	not shown	£2.74	£18.50
Bolvidon tab 20 mg			£2.33	£15.73
Norval tab 20 mg			£2.61	£17.62
Trazodone cap 50 mg	200–300 mg	600 mg	★	★
Molipaxin cap 50 mg			£4.12	£37.08
Less sedative				
Imipramine 25 mg	50–100 mg	200 mg	£0.14	£0.84
Tofranil 25 mg			£0.63	£3.78
Clomipramine cap 25 mg	30–50 mg	250 mg	£1.29	£3.87
Anafranil cap 25 mg			£1.29	£3.87
Lofepramine	140–210 mg	not shown	★	★
Gamanil 70 mg			£3.56	£16.02
Serotonin uptake inhibitors				
Fluoxetine	20 mg	20 mg	★	★
Prozac cap 20 mg			£21.37	£32.05
Paroxetine	20 mg	50 mg	★	★
Seroxat tab 20 mg			£22.60	£33.90
Sertraline	50–100 mg	200 mg	★	★
Lustral tab 50 mg			£18.95	£56.82
Fluvoxamine	100–200 mg	300 mg	★	★
Faverin tab 50 mg			£8.33	£49.98
MAO inhibitors				
Phenelzine	15–45 mg	60 mg	★	★
Nardil 15 mg			£1.33	£5.99
Tranylcypromine	10 mg	30 mg	★	★
Parnate tab 10 mg			£0.91	£1.37
Other antidepressants				
Flupenthixol	1–2 mg	3 mg	★	★
Fluanxol tab 1 mg			£2.39	£7.17
Lithium carbonate	★★	★★	★	★
Camcolit tab 250 mg			£0.59	★
Liskonum tab 450 mg			£0.94	★
Phasal tab 300 mg			£1.27	★
Priadel tab 200 mg			£0.42	★

★Not available.

★★Dosage: Initially 0.25–2.0 g daily to achieve plasma concentration of 0.6–1.2 mmol/L 12 hours after preceding dose.

Source: British Medical Association and Pharmaceutical Society of Great Britain (1992) *British National Formulary.* London, BMA and Pharmaceutical Press.

Useful addresses

Association for Post-Natal Illness
25 Jerdan Place
Fulham
London SW6 1EA

A nationwide support scheme for those with postnatal depression.

The British Association for Counselling
37a Sheep Street
Rugby
Warwickshire CV21 3BX

Information on counselling organizations and trained counsellors in your area.

Carers National Association
29 Chilworth Mews
London W2 2RG

Can put carers in touch with other carers to share experiences.

Cruse Bereavement Care — *Inverness.*
Cruse House   *713741*
126 Sheen Road
Richmond
Surrey TW9 1UR

Helps anyone who has been bereaved through counselling, advice, and opportunities for social contact.

Depressives Anonymous
36 Chestnut Avenue
Beverley
North Humberside HU17 9QU
Tel: 0482-860619

Depressives Associated
PO BOX 5
Castle Town
Portland
Dorset DT5 1BQ
Tel: 081-760-0544

Information and support groups for people who suffer from depression and for relatives who want to help. Newsletter and pen-friend scheme.

Manic Depressive Fellowship
13 Rosslyn Road
Twickenham, Middlesex TW1 2AR
Tel: 081-892-2811

Local self-help groups, pen-friendship scheme, newsletter; quarterly open meetings in London.

Northern Ireland Association for Mental Health
80 University Street
Belfast BT7 1HE

Information and advice on mental health problems as well as promoting good mental health.

Relate (National Marriage Guidance)
Herbert Grey College
Little Church Street
Rugby CV21 3AP

Gives advice and counselling on relationship problems and advises on your nearest centre or look under 'R' in your telephone directory.

Royal College of Psychiatrists
17 Belgrave Square
London SW1X 8PG

Leaflets available on depression and anxiety/ phobias.

SAD Association
51 Bracewell Road
London W10 6AF

Offers support and advice to those suffering from Seasonal Affective Disorder.

The Samaritans

Offers helplines for anyone in need of a listening ear. Look under 'S' in the telephone directory for your local helpline.

Scottish Association for Mental Health
Atlantic House
38 Gardner's Crescent
Edinburgh EH3 8DQ

Leaflets and information available on all aspects of depression.

Relaxation techniques

Cassettte tapes demonstrating relaxation techniques are now commonly used by clinical psychologists for anxiety states and phobic anxiety. They can be used with benefit in depressed patients with marked anxiety symptoms and such tapes can usually be obtained from a department of clinical psychology or through a community psychiatric nurse.

For best results the doctor should demonstrate the use of the tape to the patient or arrange for this to be done by the attached community psychiatric nurse who can also do a follow-up visit to check that the tape is being used properly.

Relaxation has a long history in medicine. It is widely taught to pregnant mothers and has also been used to help cope with uncomfortable procedures in hospital or in dentistry. Some health centres now have relaxation sessions for anxious or phobic patients, often run by a clinical psychologist or community psychiatric nurse.

People who practise meditation or yoga exercises use relaxation as part of the process. There is considerable research evidence that relaxation has beneficial physical as well as psychological effects. The physiological changes which take place during relaxation are associated with a decrease in sympathetic activity. Marked sympathetic over-activity gives rise to symptoms of anxiety and panic. Deep relaxation significantly reduces skeletal muscle tone which can bring about relief from tension, headaches, backache and other common aches and pains. The relaxation response has also been shown to decrease heart and respiratory rate and also blood pressure.

EEG tracings taken during a relaxation exercise show intensification of alpha wave activity. In anxiety states alpha wave activity is notably absent. These changes brought about by the relaxation response are distinct from those observed when sitting quietly at rest or during sleep.

The following explanation and instructions can be given to the patient as an aide mémoire after demonstrating the tape.

Relax

Anxiety is the opposite of relaxation and teaching yourself to relax reduces tension and helps to prevent it returning. Relaxation is a skill like learning to ride a bicycle – it does need practice.

Most people who are suffering from tension also suffer a loss of confidence. Some may also begin to worry that they will never recover and start each day by worrying over how they feel and each symptom is met by increased despair. Recovery is gradual and your nervous system will need time to return to its previous state. After all, even after a physical illness it takes many weeks to recover fully, even when the original infection has passed. So don't measure your progress from day to day and don't become obsessed with your symptoms. Take each day as it comes and concentrate on that day rather than what is going on inside you.

It is quite usual for a person who is recovering to feel that they have overcome the problems only to have a few bad days. Don't be put off by this. Your system, particularly during recovery will go up and down and often this is a sign of improvement rather than a cause for despair. Treat a bad day as a further chance to practise your skills at coping and don't worry, you are not slipping back.

Preparation for the relaxation exercise

1. Use a quiet room where noise levels are low and where you will not be disturbed. Ensure that you are on your own.

2. Check that you are comfortable. If you are too cold, your muscles will not relax. If you are too hot, you will be too uncomfortable to concen-

trate properly. Avoid tight clothing. Take off your shoes and spectacles.

3. Close your eyes during the relaxation to aid concentration. A darkened room also helps.

4. Allow at least half an hour during which to practise relaxation. Do not hurry yourself, or you will not relax properly.

5. Initially, when you are learning the exercises, practise them when you are feeling relatively calm. Your concentration will be better then. Later when you are better at relaxing you can use relaxation to calm yourself down if you become very tense and irritable.

6. Try to practise the exercises twice daily. If this is inconvenient, aim for at least once a day. Practise before going to bed. Sleep usually improves as a result of this.

7. Practise the exercises in a comfortable easy chair with a high back so that your head is supported. Alternatively try them lying on the floor with a cushion under your head or on your bed. When you become more skilled, practise the exercises in different settings.

How relaxation feels

As you begin to relax, the muscle group you are concentrating on will start to feel pleasantly heavy. You may also experience sensations of warmth or tingling. As your muscles become more profoundly relaxed, this sensation of heaviness will give way to a light floating feeling, during which you may lose the sensation of the bed or chair underneath you. This indicates an excellent relaxation response. At a mental level, you are likely to feel drowsy, but at the same time you are aware of your surroundings and experience a pleasant sense of calmness and well being.

Points to remember when using your relaxation tape:

1. Remember that learning to relax is like learning any new skill. It takes time. Do not expect too much in the initial stages.

2. Adopt a passive attitude. Just let relaxation happen. Progress at your own pace and avoid trying to force it.

3. Avoid worrying about whether you are relaxing properly. This will interfere with your concentration.

4. You may have distracting thoughts during practice. This is a common occurrence. Do not worry about them, accept them, push them away gently and return to attending to the relaxation commentary.

5. You may experience unfamiliar sensations such as tingling in your fingers or feelings of floating and sometimes losing control. These happen because you have been unable to relax for so long. These sensations will become less disturbing with regular relaxation practice. Remind yourself that as you learn to let go of your muscle tension, you will achieve a greater degree of control over your feelings.

Further reading

Mainly for doctors

Edwards H (1987) *Psychological Problems: Who can help?* Leicester, British Psychological Society.

Kelly D and France R (1987) *A Practical Handbook for the Treatment of Depression.* Carnforth, Lancashire, Parthenon.

McKeon P (1986) *Coping with Depression and Elation.* London, Sheldon Press.

Newton J (1988) *Preventing Mental Illness.* London, Routledge.

Royal College of General Practitioners (1987) *The Presentation of Depression: Current Approaches. Occasional Paper 36.* London, RCGP.

Mainly for patients

Berryman J et al. (1991) *Psychology and You: an Informal Introduction.* Leicester, British Psychological Society.

Blackburn I (1992) *Coping with Depression.* Edinburgh, Chambers.

Charlesworth E and Nathan R (1987) *Stress Management: a Comprehensive Guide to Your Wellbeing.* London, Corgi.

Gillet R (1987) *Overcoming Depression.* London, Dorling Kindersley.

Jacques P (1987) *Understanding Children's Problems: Helping Families to Help Themselves.* London, Unwin.

Kuipers L and Bobbington P (1987) *Living with Mental Illness.* London, Souvenir Press.

Lake T (1987) *Defeating Depression.* Harmondsworth, Penguin.

McKeon P (1986) *Coping with Depression and Elation.* London, Sheldon Press.

Orford J (1987) *Coping with Disorder in the Family.* London and Sydney, Croom Helm.

Rush J (1983) *Beating Depression.* London, Century Publishing.

Watts M (1980) *Defeating Depression.* London, Thorsons.

Winter R (1985) *The Roots of Sorrow: Reflections on Depression and Hope.* Basingstoke, Marshalls.

Diary of a depressed patient over Christmas

10 December 1984

16.25 hours

I feel that I must now terminate my employment. I don't know how long I'm going to be here. I feel that my employer has done enough for me. I can't this time accept help on an indefinité basis. I must resign and allow him to get some more permanent help. I feel guilty sitting here and being paid, after having been paid for the five months I had off earlier this year.

It probably seems a very silly thing to say, but I also feel that I've overstretched my entitlement to help from the NHS. What I mean is, that I feel that the contributions I have paid over the years I have been working have already been spent in my previous stay. I know the argument of saying that in the future I'll be making contributions to pay for the current time in hospital, but I don't know what or how long my future will last and everything has to be paid for!

What it boils down to is I feel I'm wasting people's time. When I look at some of the older men here I wish I could change places with them. They somehow seem so full of life that they could live it again, whilst I can't see anything to make it worth while, so I might as well be the age some of these men are. At least death by natural causes would be that much closer.

20.22 hours

What's the point in all this! I can't see one at all at the moment. Without the hope of a positive outcome, why stay here!

12 December 1984

11.15 hours

A little uptight just now. I don't know if I want to see any visitors today or not. I feel as though everyone is looking at me, criticizing me. I still have this feeling I'm wasting people's time that might be put to better use elsewhere. I feel guilty because I feel this way. It would solve a lot of problems if I wasn't here.

I struggled to write that bit because there is the possibility that someone will read this. I could quite easily make life easier for others if I just was not here.

A lot of people when they ask how you are feeling don't really want to know your real feelings. That has turned into a courtesy question with an almost rhetorical answer of ambiguity as the usual response.

I don't know if there is much point staying here, yet I don't think I'll find help anywhere else.

I'm treating this as a record which may be looked at later either by myself or some other. I'm doing basically the same with my cameras – making a record of how I feel and how I see things. I have no confidence of a future at all.

Coming back here in itself was admitting defeat. I can imagine the friction and tension and worry I must be causing my parents and family by being here in this state. That could be corrected quite easily, then perhaps they could get back to normal.

12.25 hours

People's attempts at reassurance just wash over me like the tide on the rocks, it does not alter them.

T.L. thinks he might get out today, he's happy but I don't think he will. I can't imagine myself in that position just now. I couldn't cope with that.

13 December 1984

19.23 hours

My moods seem to go from extreme to extreme very quickly. As mentioned earlier I felt pretty good this afternoon, happy with my progress, then it just seems to crumble. With things happening like this it's difficult for me to be sure of the progress that some of the nurses tell me I'm making.

It's just like being lifted high then having someone take the support away. In a way it's almost as bad as being continually depressed. Everyone seems to be getting gee'd up for Christmas: the radio; the TV; in the wards; but it's just not doing anything for me. I can't settle for that, I can't find any enthusiasm.

I wonder if people think I'm feigning and faking. Maybe because I'm not that good at communicating with people, they think maybe that I'm false. If they do I'm sorry.

Honestly, right now I feel I could kill myself. Life is poor right now so no-one will really miss me for long. There is nothing worth living for. I don't see the situation changing either. So what is the point in being here?

I'm sorry I haven't made much impression on the world, I haven't had much to give and I don't have any more left.

I have no hope of a permanent cure. If, I say, if I survive this one, the situation will just repeat itself under slightly different circumstances and what would be the point of reliving this again. None, it's futile. Life is futile. The world would be better off with one less unhappy individual in it. All I seem to have managed to do is create concern and I don't want anyone to be anxious or concerned or to worry over me at all.

15 December 1984

21.50 hours

I've struggled through nearly 28 years, I don't want to do the same again, I won't do the same. Twenty-eight like this past year would not be worth it. I'd rather cash the chips in now. The time grows closer.

16 December 1984

11.45 hours

The desolation feeling of last night has eased a bit this morning. I have this feeling of unworthiness and wonder at times why I am here. The fear of the treatment and stay here being unsuccessful hangs heavy on me. I sometimes get myself really tied in knots trying to do a self analysis. Usually I end up giving it a miss because of the depression it causes.

In fact, if you catalogued my life I'm sure it would end up as just one long list of failures. I'm sure that I don't want to let that situation continue much longer.

17 December 1984

17.50 hours

So far so good, no down swing so far. It's a little disconcerting after so long with swings to actually be stable for a while. It's something I could get used to.

21 December 1984

14.37 hours

All the same this will be a Christmas unlike any other I have experienced. It's difficult to pin down and identify my feelings; apprehension would be one of the main items but also the thought strikes that I would rather have my family not visit on Christmas day, but rather that they meet and be merry and not worry about me. I would survive for that small a time.

22 December 1984

18.44 hours

I've just come from having a chat with A: I asked him if he could say that he has seen any improvement in me. I sometimes do see what can be an improvement but when the swings come they can be so deep that I begin to question whether I actually did have the good days. Life prospects don't look too good at the present time.

25 December 1984

13.05 hours

Merry Christmas! That is echoed all round the hospital and more particularly, our wing. Yet though I have returned the greeting, it has not been with any conviction. As I've said before I have no enthusiasm for Christmas this year. I feel unworthy of being included in Christmas festivities because of this. At this moment in time, Christmas leaves me cold. Whilst I show this lack of interest, I cannot and should not be included in the festival.

I'll feel guilty and embarrassed when my visitors arrive, if I'm not able to put on a face; that's saying if my face reflects some joviality it will be a fake. A person who is not sure of his own life or is considering taking his own life cannot expect to be included in the festivities.

19.18 hours

I managed to fake my way through visiting time today. I painted a brighter picture than what is true. I wonder just how many people know to what extent my depression goes?

Life just now seems to be one big deception and I am growing weary of it. Treatment at the hospital does not really seem to be making much of an impression on me. Granted there is some improvement during the EC treatment, but we are only talking in periods just over 24 hours.

26 December 1984

10.13 hours

It's a beautiful day but most of it is just washing over me. I know I should be taking the benefit of such a sunny day but because my outlook is so poor, I can't really settle to this.

It's difficult to motivate myself to do anything at all at the moment. I don't know if this is an effect of some of the tablets I'm taking or whether it is just my furthering lack of enthusiasm for life. This is really beginning to bother me. I feel so utterly helpless. It's not like having a cold and taking an aspirin to clear it. I can do nothing. When you feel that way it's all too easy to slip down and lose hope.

13.50 hours

I feel guilty about not being able to switch on to the Christmas atmosphere. I am embarrassed by the fact that people around me seem to be enjoying the event. My parents and relations brought several presents up yesterday and I could only reply with a box of chocolates. I felt a sense of guilt and shame. Shame for initially having to spend time in here; shame for feeling the way I do but not being able to do anything about it.

28 December 1984

21.00 hours

I'm as jittery as hell, with and without the shake. I find it extremely difficult to persuade myself that

I'm worth staying alive. I look at myself and see all that is bad: I'm here requiring treatment; but not for the first time, this is the second. I can only see myself back here again, but I can't see that as beneficial to myself so there is no point. It's another thing I have failed in. I don't think I could name one activity that I could say I have succeeded in doing well.

I even feel guilty about people coming up here to visit me. I can't justify it. I don't warrant the time spent.

I really don't see any hope of finally getting better, so without hope it would be much more sensible to bring to a close the life that in the present is only making a burden of itself to my parents, friends, relations and not least the staff here at the hospital.

I see futile attempts at suicide here which only strengthens the resolve to make especially sure that my attempt will be wholly successful. 'Attempt' is not the word to use, I don't know the word I'm looking for.

29 December 1984

16.23 hours

I'm sitting here just wondering how much longer I'll permit this to continue. I feel guilty for taking up people's time. This existence would be better terminated. I'd cause less bother to die than for the nurses to spend time looking after what I consider to be a lost cause.

My bank balance and building society accounts should now cover any debts on my bike and also cover my funeral costs. I have no other major debts that I can think of. Not quite true – Marks and Spencer account card, but there should be enough to cover that as well.

19.57 hours

There is no point in continuing with this charade! I am doing nothing more than wasting people's time. I'm sorry, I'm really sorry! I'm only a waster, useless, of no worth to anyone. I'm sorry for the time of nurses, doctors, and everybody else's time that I've wasted. I thought for a while that I could get through this, that a cure might be possible but now I see that won't be possible. If I were to get through this crisis and get back out to the outside world, another crisis would soon loom and it would come to the same climax except that it would be played to completion. So what is the point of delaying fate? None. Quite blankly none. Jesus Christ, I hate myself! Let me seek death, in whatever means I can find, in peace.

30 December 1984

22.16 hours

Just watched the last half hour of "Kramer versus Kramer". It looks from what I saw that it was an excellent film. It shows a point which is relevant to me. Basically I'm frightened to get involved in relationships in case they go wrong, in case they failed, in case I failed. I fear what the film portrayed. Not so much for my benefit, but I don't want to hurt someone else, not anybody else, by wrongful action on my part. I don't want to hurt anyone.

31 December 1984

13.53 hours

The last day of the year! Well I've got a lot further than I was expecting!

1 January 1985

21.23 hours

I've had a good day, that's two in a row! It's a pleasant sensation but it's almost as though I feel guilty about not feeling bad. I told the folks of my realization as written in the previous entry. They seemed to take this as a good sign. I hope it is too but I don't want them to read too much into it; I've still got a long way to go.

I managed to get Dad worked into a game of cribbage with Uncle T's help. It was good, at least he got the basics. Perhaps a game for the future.

I'm enjoying a Villiger cigar whilst writing this entry, along with a can of shandy.

Again it doesn't seem like a New Year's Day. Noise is blowing from the television yet I feel cut off from it by immersing myself in writing what I have called my diary.

8 January 1985

10.39 hours

I feel a bit on the nervous side this morning. For a long time I've just let the days slip by, not thinking of work or really of life, at all. Now I find myself thinking of work and if I'm able to cope with it. Or thinking about how I could live if I did not have a job at all! I also at times think ahead to the time when I come off these drugs and whether I'll slip back into depression. These thoughts don't do me any good at all, even now. I'm not really very happy.

It's a bit distressing because I have been quite relaxed for a reasonable time but now all the doubts are back.

10 January 1985

13.01 hours

It's ridiculous, if there is an argument or difference of opinion, between any two other parties, I feel that in some way, I'm to blame. I feel guilty in some respect.

12 January 1985

07.45 hours

I can't give my parents what they want to hear, that I'm feeling better. It would be a lie to tell them so. I always seem to run away or avoid tense situations. I'm sitting here in the ward, alone. I'm not needed in the day room, I would just be in the way.

Despite talking with the night staff last night, I still feel I didn't get my point over. I'm trying to seek for some crumb of hope but honestly cannot find one.

14 January 1985

16.01 hours

The song, "I'll be Loving You Always", has just been on the television. The 'always' bit worries me. This suggests a long time, yet there are people who feel that they can't handle the long term, and who have serious doubts about the short term.

I have no long term hopes and I have very little short term hopes, at the moment I don't see the situation improving at all. I feel down.

When I feel down I'm more susceptible to emotional influences. What I mean is, a record will bring tears to my eyes, or a picture will or a sad scene on the television. It's a fight to prevent the tears flowing. I feel I join in the sorrow and it affects me to the bottom of my heart. It rocks me; I see the time when I will not be here.

15 January 1985

22.18 hours

The downer lasted a couple of hours, then lifted. I'm trying to find a way of explaining this. I'm content; I feel at ease! Earlier when my parents were here, I felt happy! This is even harder to explain. I feel nervous about feeling good, I even feel guilty about this. It's confusing me a little.

I'm a lot scared of it just disappearing. For so long I've been unhappy, and it's a little difficult to believe that I'm better. This must all seem pretty uninteresting to anyone else. I'm sorry for that, there is so much more to say but I don't want to be disappointed so I'll save the rest for later.

Index